MW00909298

$\mathscr{F}$ORMULAS

FOR Healthful Living

BOOKS BY FRANCIS BRINKER, N.D.

The Toxicology of Botanical Medicine

The Eclectic Dispensatory of Botanical
Therapeutics, Vol. II

FORMULAS

FOR Healthful Living

Francis Brinker, N.D.

Eclectic Medical Publications
Sandy, Oregon

Individuals with serious health problems need to be under the care of a physician. The information provided in this book is not intended to take the place of appropriate treatments provided by one's doctor.

Copyright © 1995 by Francis Brinker, N.D.
All rights reserved.

For information about permission to reproduce selections from this book, write to:
Permissions
Eclectic Medical Publications
P.O. Box 936
Sandy, Oregon 97055

Printed in the USA
ISBN 1-888483-00-8 paperback
Library of Congress Catalog Card Number:
95-83568
Edited by Kathryn Rosson
Book design by Nancy Stodart
Cover design by Richard Stodart

To Wade Boyle, N.D., whose writings and association with the naturopathic profession and botanical medicine has enriched the natural healing legacy, and whose friendship and help in my own writing endeavors has enriched my life.

❖

I would like to express appreciation and thanks for all the naturopathic doctors who instructed and endowed me with one of life's finest treasures, the knowledge of how to obtain and maintain good health. I am also indebted to fellow students who, in striving to understand, posed questions and ideas that enriched my own understanding. I am grateful for all who, having tested information and theories about health in their own experience, share their discoveries with others. To all those whose love for people and plants has led them to search for healing virtues in herbs, and to those who have worked to bring the fruits of these labors to others, I am truly grateful.

Deserving special recognition are Michael Ancharski, N.D., and David Lytle for their work on the herbal formulas in this book.

More precious than gold is health and well-being,
contentment of spirit than coral.
No treasure greater than a healthy body;
no happiness than a joyful heart!

Book of Sirach 30:15-16

CONTENTS

PREFACE

It is important to recognize that the best way to use medicinal plants for health maintenance is to combine them with other appropriate methods. It is not enough to just use herbs or other supplements as substitutes for chemical drugs. The emphasis should be to correct the underlying conditions that cause sickness. This comprehensive philosophy of the nature of health, disease, and therapeutics distinguishes naturopathic medicine from other approaches which hold similar techniques and agents in common. Naturopathic medicine utilizes all effective forms of natural therapeutics that work together with the individual's inherent capacity for health and healing.

Naturopathic doctors teach the principles of optimizing vitality in order to avoid future disease. These principles are the most important "formulas for healthful living." While it remains necessary to provide symptomatic relief for suffering, it is even more cogent to eliminate the barriers to optimum health. In this way the healing power of nature that insures our biological well-being is given the opportunity to manifest a true cure. The simplicity of the substances and techniques recommended in this book to enhance the process of healing should not dissuade anyone from considering their use. When this type of health support is persistently employed, the effects can make a profound difference in the quality of life.

Herbal remedies hold an important place in a complete approach to health optimization. Reliable information on herbs and their constituents and activities is a necessary foundation for their appropriate uses. This text uses as its primary references books on herbs that have been selected for their sound assessment of botanical remedies. These references emphasize both clinical experience with herbal products and scientific evaluation of their activity. They were written by individuals with expertise in botanical analysis, medical examination, and the therapeutic application of plants.

King's American Dispensatory stands as the epitome of materia medica texts used early in this century when herbs were still a major part of medical practice. It was written by John Uri Lloyd, the distinguished pharmacist who helped develop many American plant remedies, and Harvey Wickes Felter, an outstanding eclectic medical doctor and educator. *The Herb Book* is a recent comprehensive review of herbs commonly employed in America and Europe. It was authored by John Lust, a nephew of the man who established naturopathic medicine in America, Benedict Lust. *Herbal Medication* provides an understanding of how nontoxic herbs work with the body's inborn ability to heal itself. This modern book by English naturopaths, A.W. Priest and L.R. Priest, also describes the uses and preparations of herbs. *Herbal Medicine* by Rudolf Fritz Weiss, a contemporary German medical doctor, presents both clinical experience and current research using herbs from Europe and from around the world. The *Eclectic Dispensatory of Botanical Therapeutics,* compiled by naturopathic pharmacist, Ed Alstat, provides important historical, clinical, and research information. My contributions to this latter book include a reference guide on the specific selection of herbs for individual patients, summaries of published studies on major herbs, their constituents and actions, and the toxicology of certain plants when given in excessive doses.

The texts mentioned above are the sources for statements regarding the therapeutic uses of the herbs included in this book. Additional observations are supported by the scientific journal articles listed in the Reference section.

Also included are a guide for determining the proper dosage of the herbal formulas according to age or weight and a glossary to explain some of the terms used to describe the forms, constituents, and activities of herbs, the physiology of the human body, and health care systems or approaches that offer alternatives to drugs and surgery.

The first section in each chapter summarizes physiological principles and therapies as taught in naturopathic medical colleges. Through clinical and personal experience I have found these principles dependable and believe that the methods discussed are both practical and effective. The charts in each chapter are given as a short synopsis to simplify the information in the chapter and make it more easily accessible.

Neither the health habits nor the herbal combinations recommended in this book are "formulas" in the strict sense of that term. For instance, the herbal combinations are not presented as recipes with exact amounts listed. There are no such ideal herbal formulas of that type that will perfectly meet the needs of all individuals. **The "formulas" consisting of both suggested lifestyle adjustments and herbal supplements as given in this text are provided to help each individual make choices for themselves and their own particular situation and condition.** While such decisions are best made in consultation with a knowledgeable holistic practitioner, this book will serve as a useful guide in considering possible options.

INTRODUCTION

Herbs And Health

Traditional Herbalism

As long as humans have inhabited the earth, plants have been an important part of their health care and maintenance. Since prehistory and continuing to our modern day, people in traditional cultures have gone out to collect plants that are useful as nourishing potherbs. This is one way of using herbs to prevent disease. Long before there were pharmacies on street corners people grew herb gardens and stored dried plants in herbal medicine cabinets. In this way they provided those things that were most useful for maintaining good health or ameliorating common ailments. Oriental spices were especially valued but were restricted to those who could afford their high cost. Some herbs and spices with fragrant aromas are thought of by many today as strictly for culinary uses or beverage teas. However, their pleasant flavors have long been recognized as making these plants desirable for both enhancing meals and counteracting digestive upsets. Many of the teas were used between meals for other internal problems or as washes or soaks to alleviate external afflictions. Poultices provided the means to apply the herbs locally for sustained effects.

Though generally applied to nonwoody plants the term "herb" came to refer to any type of plant, plant part, or plant product that is used as a remedial agent. Time-honored remedies, sometimes referred to as folk medicine, were the means by which people treated themselves when they were unable to obtain, or did not need, the services of a physician. Through the ages many of the herbs used in folk medicine were also prescribed by doctors for similar purposes. Physicians generally used formulations of multiple herbs with higher potencies. From before the time of Hippocrates alcoholic beverages rather than water were preferred by physicians to extract and preserve the active principles from herbs. Distilled alcohol became more commonly used as a solvent for extraction since the Renaissance. Tinctures made with distilled alcohol continue to provide reliable products that are easily administered. Distilling herbal essential oils became popular after the 16th century and provided an importance means for producing concentrated aromatic constituents for use. Fluid extracts were developed in the 19th century to provide concentrated and standardized alcoholic extracts. While dried, powdered herbs in tablets or capsules are now commonly available, many herbal practitioners prefer using either alcoholic extracts or teas, depending on the circumstances. Ointments and creams are now the forms commonly used for topical applications.

Development of Medical Alternatives

When symptoms of deficiencies, illness, or disease arose in the past, bed rest and home remedies were usually relied upon. These remedies typically consisted of common household substances, water, foods, and herbs. Vitamin and mineral compounds were supplied by using whole foods and nutrient herbs. The usefulness of concentrated sources of specific nutrients was not understood until their recent discoveries and isolation. Medicinal herbs were given based on their activity or association with a particular organ. Recent identification of active components of herbal remedies has allowed their effects to be better understood and their application to be more specific. Vitamins, minerals, and herbs are now commonly accepted as important supplemental agents in striving to establish and maintain good health. Laboratory and clinical research support this development. In the process the usefulness of many folk medicines has been substantiated. However, many of these available means to better health have not gained acceptance by those who dictate conventional medical practice.

The emphasis in conventional medicine has always been on powerful, toxic drugs to counteract disease symptoms and surgical intervention to excise diseased or damaged tissue. Most of the professions that specialize in using techniques or substances other than surgery or drugs arose in response to the need for medical reform. Such was the case in the 19th century with American contributions to the development of physiomedicalism (medical herbalism), homeopathy, hygienics, hydrotherapy, physiotherapy, and chiropractic. Many of these practices struggled to survive due in large part to propaganda and political opposition from mainstream medicine. The founders of eclectic medicine and osteopathy incorporated some of these approaches into their practices while continuing to utilize surgery and drugs.

The Role of Naturopathic Medicine

At the beginning of the 20th century influence from European reformers helped transform the remaining American drugless movements into a complete system of natural health care. This system became known as naturopathic medicine. The naturopathic profession has kept abreast of modern developments in the scientific understanding of medicine. At the same time it has continued to rely on physiologic curative principles and therapeutic agents and techniques that find their source in nature. The empirical art of herbal medicine is studied and its basis in pharmacological science is kept up to date as part of the naturopathic understanding and approach.

The importance of disease prevention, always a major emphasis of naturopathy, is being recognized more in our current concept of medicine. The general public continues to seek information on ways to improve health which are safe, effective, and available at low cost. People are paying greater attention to their diets. Many health-conscious individuals use dietary supplements to insure they meet the demands caused by the stresses of modern life. Exercise programs have gained in popularity. Hatha yoga, t'ai chi ch'uan, and other relaxation and movement techniques that help balance mental and physical activity enjoy increasing participation. The modern focus on nutrition and exercise has led to an abundance of new health food stores, natural foods groceries, health clubs, fitness centers, and martial arts training facilities in some communities. Renewed involvement in meditation and prayer form part of a spiritual awakening process that has resulted in health benefits for many. Awareness of the interrelatedness of a person's mental/emotional/physical health has popularized therapeutic approaches involving the entire person. In addition to the recent upsurge of attention given to the integrated naturopathic system of health care, interest in chiropractors, acupuncturists, homeopaths, nutritional counselors, massage therapists, physical therapists, biofeedback practitioners, hypnotherapists and other specialists has likewise soared. In this climate the use of herbs and their extracts is also making a comeback.

Comprehensive Health Care

The use of herbs alone does not insure the development of perfect health. Using herbal combinations is one of a number of ways to enable the body to optimize its functioning. Health involves an entire lifestyle that is attuned to the demands, or laws, of nature. The goal of complete health will elude a person's grasp unless the decision is also made to live in a way that addresses physiological, psychological, social, and spiritual needs. Information given by a physician to the patient about a particular impaired organ or system and how different choices and behaviors will impact its function is vital. However, it will prove to be advantageous to patients only if they apply the knowledge to their lives. The more a person recognizes the importance of supportive habits and incorporates these into the approach to his or her problem, the more effective the use of herbal therapy or any other method will be at improving the condition.

Conditions that are unmanageable through basic home care always require the attention of a doctor. To assure that a potentially serious condition is properly assessed, particularly any problem involving a vital organ, a diagnosis by a licensed physician is necessary. Herbal remedies are not always appropriate to replace conventional medication but can often

complement the effects of necessary drugs. Herbs
may reduce the need for high doses of drugs and in
this way alleviate the toxic side effects frequently
associated with their use. Consultation with the
attending physician is required if any change in
medication is considered. Licensed naturopathic
doctors and trained holistic physicians are best able
to advise patients on the appropriate inclusion of
natural therapeutics into one's health care regimen.

When using herbs it is important to recognize
their limitations in some cases. They are not the
complete answer for all problems. They can also
pose a danger if used too frequently or in amounts
that are too large. Greater care is required when
medical conditions other than the one that the herbs
are intended to help are also present, or when other
medications are being used. These might contraindi-
cate the use of certain herbal remedies. Consultation
with doctors or other experts with greater knowledge
is important in cases where there are serious questions about safety or incompatibilities. This applies
to any approach to health and disease including the
use of plants or their extracts.

Formulating Herbal Remedies

An herbal combination given by a naturopathic
physician or other competent herbal prescriber is
ideally formulated to specifically address the com-
plaint of the individual seeking help. In-depth
training results in the herbs being selected according
to the need for a particular form to be administered,
the activity of the herb and its constituents and, in the
case of naturopathic or holistic doctors, the underlying causes and development of the condition. Herbal
therapy is most effective when the remedy is formulated for a particular individual, since each person

presents their own unique characteristics and requirements that contribute to their problem and to its
resolution. The training of a licensed physician
allows them to more thoroughly evaluate a patient
based upon the findings of their medical and case
history, physical examination, laboratory tests, and
thorough case analysis. The herbs that are most
appropriate to resolve the condition and relieve the
symptoms of that particular patient are then chosen
over other similar plants. Several plants or their
extracts are usually combined to produce the desired
effect in a balanced fashion. What one component
lacks another will provide, so that the combined
action improves what is accomplished by a single
herb. While some herbs in the remedy may relieve
symptoms, others can act to correct their cause.
Exact instructions on using the formula to assure the
best results are given to the patient. Such a prescription can then be adjusted to accommodate the
changes that occur as a result of the overall therapy.
Unfortunately, in many places there is no one sufficiently adept to tailor formulas specifically to individual needs.

The herbal formulas in this book are presented
under the premise that it is possible to achieve desirable results from a standard combination of herbs
since there is often a commonality to problems that
affect a particular system of the body. Such combinations can prove beneficial even though they are not
designed specifically for an individual but address a
general condition. Though sometimes denigrated as a
"shotgun" approach to illness, combining herbs in
this manner is effective when the functions of a
particular system are supported and/or improved.
Sometimes using two complementary formulas or
"giving it both barrels" is preferable. The latter

approach can achieve the desired purpose better than a single formula when there are several organ systems or interdependent problems needing correction. It is always important to use at least one formula that addresses the underlying cause and not just the typical symptoms of a condition. Otherwise, there will be no long lasting results or true benefit.

The herbal formulations presented here are designed to give broad support or enhancement to particular organ functions. Individual extracts may be combined in appropriate proportions to produce the formula in whole or in part. Greater or lesser amounts of each herb presented in a formula can be used in order to personally adjust the desired influence. Since the formulas were designed to address necessary considerations and the herbs were selected with their complementary effects in mind, using the complete combination would be most preferable. Commercial preparations already combining the herbs in standard proportions can be used to help simplify the process.

In certain cases that are noted, glycerin is a useful additive for its own soothing and sweetening effects. The formula for use in the ear combines glycerin with olive oil extracts of certain herbs. Otherwise, alcoholic extracts are the form normally indicated. In some formulas a certain herb is indicated as having components that are best extracted with water rather than alcohol. In these cases the formula could well be taken in a tea prepared from that particular herb.

Guidelines For Using Herbal Extracts

As the nutritional requirements of individuals vary, so does their response to the action of nontoxic herbal remedies. Therefore a dosage range is the best way to discuss their use. For most formulas general guideline for an adult weighing about 150 pounds would be from 15 - 30 drops per dose taken 3 - 5 times each day. This dosage range should be applied to the formulas described herein unless otherwise noted. It is usually advisable to begin near the lower level of the dosage range and to gradually increase it until the maximum is reached or the desired effect is attained. In acute conditions it is better to take smaller doses more frequently. For example, 10 drops taken every two hours from rising until bed-time would be approximately equivalent to 30 drops taken three times per day. The total daily dose for acute conditions is generally higher than the dose taken regularly for chronic conditions. In chronic cases the practice is to rest periodically from taking the same herbs when possible. Abstaining from their use for one day per week or one weekend per month can help to prevent dependency. This also allows the body to maintain its sensitivity to the effects of the herbs. Of course, if the function of a vital organ such as the heart or lungs is being supported, sudden discontinuation of herbs or other types of medication is inadvisable. Some remedies can become toxic by taking too much or by using them for too long. The dose of an herb used as part of a formula is generally less than its dose would be if it were taken alone. In the same way when combining formulas lower doses for each formula are usually appropriate due to their complementary or synergistic effects.

The proper dosage of herbal extract combinations also varies between individuals. Even when an herbal supplement is standardized to contain a certain amount of some active constituent, the effect will depend on the sensitivity of the person using it. Besides the nature of the condition being treated, the initial dosage is based on constitutional strength, weight, and age. In general large, robust individuals require larger doses than those who are small and frail. Some women tend to need a smaller dose than men of the same size. For those over the age of 60 smaller doses are necessary except for some laxatives and diuretics which may need to be given in larger than normal amounts. For infants and children and those who weigh much less than a normal adult (about 150 lbs.) special rules (Young's, Cowling's, and Clark's - see Dosage Adjustments) are used to determine the proper reduction in dosage. Clark's rule also provides the correct dosage increase for those who weigh much more than 150 pounds (about 70 kg).

Liquid herbal extracts are easier to swallow than capsules or tablets. The active components are readily absorbed in the gut because they are already in solution. By simply varying the number of drops used the dosage can be increased or reduced precisely according to the need. These extracts are more concentrated than a typical beverage tea so drinking large amounts of fluids is not required. They can be taken in a small amount of water or other liquid. If added to an appropriate warm herbal tea the effect can be supported and absorption improved. Extracts containing alkaloidal constituents should not be consumed together with regular black tea, since the tannins in this tea precipitate the alkaloids and reduce their absorption. Liquid extracts may also be added to a favorite juice. Grape juice is one of the best at disguising strong flavors. Unless the herbal extracts are being used to influence digestion, it is generally preferable to take them between meals to optimize absorption.

The following chapters are designed to introduce principles for optimizing health. The herbal formulas presented describe the qualities of the herbs and their relationship to particular bodily organs and functions. The reader is encouraged to explore these herbal qualities in the context of their overall health and choose them alone or in combination to create a healthy balance in their lives.

HERBS AND OTHER THERAPIES

Home Remedies	Commercial Preparations	Self Care	Professional Care
Potherbs	Tinctures	Food	Naturopathy
Spices	Essential Oils	Water	Physio-
Teas	Fluid Extracts	Herbs	medicalism
Poultices	Tablets	Household	Homeopathy
	Capsules	Substances	Hygienics
	Ointments	Vitamins	Hydrotherapy
	Creams	Minerals	Physiotherapy
		Exercise	Chiropractic
		Rest	Osteopathy
		Relaxation	Eclectic/holistic
		Meditation	Acupuncture
		Prayer	Massage
			Biofeedback
			Hypnosis

SOME ADVANTAGES OF MEDICAL SUPERVISION BY A PHYSICIAN

Gives Complete Therapeutic Protocol
e.g., advises on lifestyle management

Assesses Seriousness Of Condition
e.g., determines vital organ involvement

Monitors Effects Of Medication
e.g., changes medical prescriptions

Determines Safe Level Of Herb Use
e.g., rules out herbal contraindications

CHOOSING HERBAL COMBINATIONS

Standard Formulations	Prescribed Individually

Conditions Recognized:
Involved Systems Identified
Symptoms Noted

Formulas Designed To:
Alleviate Symptoms
Address General Causes
Support/Enhance Functions

Formulas Produced:
Alcoholic Extracts Combined
Dosage Adjustments

Formulas Combined For:
Related Problems
Other Systems Involved

Patients Individually Assessed:
Medical History
Personal History
Physical Exam
Lab Tests
Case Analysis

Therapy Determined:
Dysfunction & Cause Identified
Specific Herbs & Forms Selected
Exact Instructions Given

Follow-up Evaluations:
Formula Changed As Needed

USING HERBAL FORMULAS

Dosage Issues	Liquid Extracts

Dosage Differs For Individuals
  And For Formulas
Begin With Low Doses
Acute Case - Low, Frequent Doses
Chronic Case - Stop Periodically
  (if herb support is not vital-too
  much or too long can be toxic)
Minimum Dose Necessary
Robust Patient - Larger Dose
Frail Patient - Smaller Dose
Children - Smaller Dose
Elderly - Smaller Dose
Over 150 lbs. - Larger Dose
Under 150 lbs. - Smaller Dose

Easier To Swallow
Easier To Absorb
Dosage Adjusted Readily
Small Volume Of Fluid To Consume
Take With Herb Tea Or Juice
Do Not Take With Black Tea
Take Between Meals

Dosage Adjustments

Normal Dosage

Unless otherwise noted, the average dose of these liquid extract formulas for an adult weighing about 150 pounds (70 kg) is 15 - 30 drops taken in a little water 3 - 5 times daily. This may be increased under directions from a physician. For children or those whose weights are significantly more or less than this, there are several rules that can be used to help estimate the proper dose.

Young's Rule

To determine the appropriate dose based on age for children, Young's rule is used. It states that for a child the fraction of the adult dose is determined by the child's age divided by the child's age plus 12. So if a child is 4 years old, the dose would be 4/16 or one fourth of the adult dose.

For example, if the Antiseptic Formula is used by an adult as a gargle for a sore throat and then swallowed in doses of 20 drops in a little water every 3 hours, a 4-year old child could use 5 drops in the same way just as frequently.

Cowling's Rule

For those from age 12 to 24 years, this rule becomes more appropriate. At these ages take the year number of the next birthday and divide by 24. For someone who will be 16 years old they would receive 16/24 or two thirds of the adult dose. Of course, after age 24 the adult dose becomes the norm.

For example, a 25-year old man's dose of the

Liver Tonic Formula taken after eating too much fried food could be 30 drops in grape juice. A soon to be 16-year old of similar size would use 20 drops instead for an equivalent effect.

Clark's Rule

Clark's rule uses weight to determine the dose. The weight of a person in pounds is divided by 150 to give the fraction of the adult dose to be used. For instance, if a 30-year old woman weighs 120 pounds she would take 120/150 or four fifths of the adult dose. If her husband were the same age and weighed 200 pounds, he would take 200/150 or one and one third the adult dose.

For example, if this couple both wanted to use the Alterative Formula as part of a prolonged cleansing regimen, a typical dose might be 30 drops three times each day. She would take 24 drops three times daily while he could take 40 drops three times or 30 drops four times each day.

I

CLEANSING & IMMUNITY

Blood And Lymph

A fundamental aspect of health is the quality of the composition of the fluids that circulate in the body. Good health requires the elimination of toxic waste and the removal of foreign substances and microbial invaders.

In the past, blood was considered synonymous with life. This concept deserves attention. It is appropriate to associate vitality with the quality of the blood. **Blood brings nourishment to the cells of our body and removes their waste.** This exchange is accomplished as the fluid in the arterial blood escapes from tiny vessels called capillaries into the space surrounding the cells of the body. The nutrients in this fluid are absorbed by the cells. The cellular waste then enters with the fluid into the venous capillary blood or returns in the lymph fluid to the venous circulation through lymph vessels. It is as important to the health of cells and tissues to remove this soluble waste as it is to provide good nutrition.

Cleansing the blood occurs as it is filtered through the emunctories (organs which excrete cellular waste products). These organs include the kidneys, liver, skin, and lungs. While the lungs expel the gases dissolved in the blood, the sweat glands of the skin excrete some mineral salts and other soluble substances. The kidneys excrete most of the soluble waste from the blood. However, it is necessary for certain compounds to be processed by the liver before they can be excreted in the urine. If the liver does not adequately metabolize (chemically change) ammonia, bilirubin, or certain steroids these compounds accumulate and produce toxic symptoms. Drugs and other toxins from outside the body are also metabolized in the liver. The liver excretes some of the changed waste products into the intestines in the bile. These metabolized compounds are normally eliminated through the colon along with the waste from undigested food.

In cases of constipation the reabsorption of some of these waste compounds from the colon contaminates the blood. Toxins produced by intestinal bacteria from the breakdown of undigested protein can also be absorbed. An increased burden of waste excretion then falls on the skin, lungs, and kidneys as toxins accumulate in the blood. If their elimination is inadequate, symptoms such as skin rashes or blemishes, bad breath, foul-smelling gas, or dark, concentrated urine typically result. **When the emunctories do not function adequately, waste accumulates in the blood and becomes increasingly difficult to remove effectively from around the cells.** These compounds poison the tissues throughout the body as cells become enveloped in toxins. This in turn aggravates previously existing health problems.

By regularly employing methods of active sweating, deep breathing, and generous fluid consumption the emunctories are given most of the means to function properly. Regular vigorous exercise is an ideal way of helping assure that these needs are met. Maintaining optimal blood purification especially requires efficient bowel function. Optimal elimination from the bowels is aided by exercise, proper fluid intake, and dietary fiber from whole foods. Keeping the blood purified is further promoted by reducing exposure to outside toxins such as drugs, pollutants, and food contaminants. Intensive cleansing regimens such as scientific fasting, colonic irrigation, and constitutional hydrotherapy are extremely helpful for the cleansing necessary in chronic conditions. The results of these procedures can be dramatic in severe cases. **Herbs that increase different excretory activities are especially indicated for chronic elimination problems.**

While the cells in the blood are mostly red blood cells for carrying oxygen to the tissues and removing carbon dioxide, the function of the less numerous white blood cells is not so simple. Some white blood cells from the spleen and bone marrow act as scavengers in the blood. **Besides circulating in the blood, scavenger cells are found in the body's tissues (especially in the lungs, liver, spleen, thymus, and lymph nodes) and lymph fluid. They destroy microbes (bacteria, viruses, yeast, and protozoa) by phagocytosis (ingestion or consumption) and remove dead tissue, foreign cells, and other unwanted material.** Other types of white blood cells produce antibodies or work with the scavengers as part of the inflammatory reaction. Together these cells make up our immune system. They work on both fluid and cellular levels to cleanse the blood and tissues of allergens, infections, and mutations. Since this immune activity produces waste products, the cleansing measures that improve elimination are an associated function.

Different methods are used to optimize immunity. Hygienic practices such as washing, proper food preparation, and appropriate poison and waste disposal reduce bacterial and toxin exposure and lessen the demands upon the immune system. Avoiding foods or air-born substances that produce allergic sensitivities can be a critical factor in overcoming chronic conditions that may appear unrelated to allergies. Techniques that help manage stress also indirectly support the immune response. Exercise, massage, and hydrotherapy are beneficial physical factors since pressure from muscular contraction and movement enhances the circulation of the blood and lymph. Nutritional supplements that enhance immune activity include vitamin C, beta-carotene, and zinc. **Herbs that stimulate phagocytosis are an important means of improving the immune response.**

Alterative Formula

The following alterative formula is similar to an extract combination that was popular circa 1900. The latter was frequently used as an alterative to help resolve rheumatic conditions and chronic infections because of its tonic and eliminative properties. A modified version was later made official by being listed in the *National Formulary* as Compound Fluidextract Trifolium. Alteratives have also been called "blood purifiers" for their gentle effects on organs that remove the metabolic waste and toxins from the circulation. They are used for prolonged periods in chronic conditions.

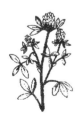

A liquid extract of **red clover** (*Trifolium pratense*) blossoms has been a favorite alterative for its effects on the lungs and liver. The flavonoid isoquercitrin is an important constituent. Water-soluble polysaccharides in a red clover extract showed antitumor effects and stimulated white blood cell accumulation. Red clover tea is a good vehicle to use for tinctures because the polysaccharides are not in the alcoholic extract.

Burdock (*Arctium lappa*) root contains polysaccharides with similar activity to those found in red clover. Burdock root's alcoholic extract has also inhibited tumor growth. A component of the root has been shown to reduce cellular mutations caused by certain chemicals. Polyacetylenes from the root have demonstrated potent antibacterial and antifungal effects. The root is valued for its alterative activity, its diaphoretic property (increases sweating), and its mild laxative effect. The arctiin and arctigenin content in burdock seeds make the seeds useful as a diuretic for kidney disorders.

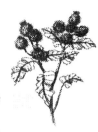

Licorice (*Glycyrrhiza glabra*) root has been used as a mild laxative and a soothing demulcent for inflamed mucous membranes of the throat, stomach, and intestines. Isoflavonoids of licorice are antimicrobial against Staph. bacteria and Candida yeast. The sweet flavor of glycyrrhizin (also called glycyrrhizic acid or glycyrrhizinic acid) in the licorice helps to mask the bitterness of other herbs. Glycyrrhizin is antiviral. It also increases interferon production which aids the immune system in protection from viral infections. The aglycone of glycyrrhizin is glycyrrhetic acid (also called glycyrrhetinic acid) which has demonstrated antitussive, anti-inflammatory, and anti-arthritic properties. It also inhibits the binding and effects of several tumor promoters. The potassium loss and water retention caused by the glycyrrhetic acid can be managed by using only small quantities of licorice in combinations and by resting periodically from its use. The potassium and diuretics in this formula also help prevent these problems. **People with signs of or a history of high blood pressure or heart failure should**

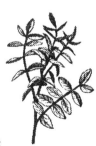

avoid using licorice regularly.

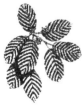

Oregon grape (*Berberis aquifolium,* also called *Mahonia aquifolium*) root has been found to be most useful as an alterative for skin problems associated with poor liver or bowel function. It has been employed as a digestive tonic, mild laxative, and diuretic. The root contains large amounts of the alkaloid berberine. Berberine is an effective antimicrobial agent against disease-causing bacteria, yeast, and protozoa. This alkaloid also inhibits diarrhea caused by bacterial bowel toxins. Berberine increases acute bilirubin output by the liver when its excretion is low and blood bilirubin levels are high. Along with other alkaloids from this plant, oxyacanthine and berbamine, berberine stimulates total biliary secretions. Berberine and jatrorrhizine, another alkaloid constituent, have anti-inflammatory activity. Berberine has shown some positive effect on inflammation of the liver caused by industrial poisons. In addition, berberine is a potent activator for white blood cells that have antitumor activity.

Buckthorn (*Rhamnus frangula*) bark is well known for its laxative properties. It does not produce tolerance nor constipating after-effects. Though it is closely related to cascara sagrada their anthracene derivatives and activity are different. **Like other laxatives it should not be used during pregnancy because it may cause reflex contractions of the uterus.**

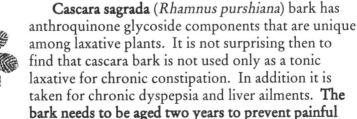

Cascara sagrada (*Rhamnus purshiana*) bark has anthroquinone glycoside components that are unique among laxative plants. It is not surprising then to find that cascara bark is not used only as a tonic laxative for chronic constipation. In addition it is taken for chronic dyspepsia and liver ailments. **The bark needs to be aged two years to prevent painful**

irritation to the bowel lining caused by use of the fresh bark.

Prickly ash (*Xanthoxylum*, or *Zanthoxylum*, *clava-herculis*) bark is considered an alterative, diaphoretic, and stimulant. It also acts as a digestive tonic. Its isobutylamide neoherculin creates a sense of warmth caused by stimulation of glandular secretions in the mouth and of mucous membranes of the gastrointestinal tract. Its lignin component asarinin is useful in kidney disorders. The alkaloid chelerythrine found in the bark is both antimicrobial and anti-inflammatory.

Queen's root (*Stillingia sylvatica*) is another alterative in this combination that stimulates secretory activity of mucous membranes. In this case it is due to the action of its diterpene esters. It was used for irritation of the throat and lungs and valued for enhancing lymphatic functions. To be of value the extract must be made from the fresh root.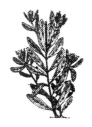

Bitter orange (*Citrus vulgaris*, also called *C. aurantium*) oil is not in itself bitter. Rather, the oil is derived from the peel of the bitter orange. Though it is typically used as a flavoring, its very high content of the terpene d-limonene has additional benefits. The oil and limonene have antiseptic effects against bacteria and fungus. Limonene also helps to prevent the development of cancer in rats and cell cultures that have been exposed to carcinogens.

Potassium iodide is a nonherbal ingredient which provides two essential nutrients. Potassium is critical for normal cellular metabolism. Its intake has diminished with the decline of vegetable consumption in the American diet. The inclusion of potassium in this formula helps to replace what might be lost through the effects of the licorice root. Iodine is essential for proper functioning of the thyroid gland which regulates the basic metabolic rate throughout the body. Potassium iodide also produces an expectorant effect by increasing the secretion of a watery fluid from the respiratory membranes. This mucosal wash helps flush out trapped particles and phlegm. **It must be noted that consuming excessive amounts of potassium iodide for a prolonged period can result in "iodism." Its symptoms can include a runny nose, sinus headache, eruptions on the skin, nausea, loss of appetite, or weakness. If any of these occur, use of the formula should be stopped until the symptoms disappear.** Its consumption can then be resumed after reducing the dosage by one half.

The combination of herbs in the alterative formula is also similar to the controversial Hoxsey tonic. The Hoxsey tonic is known for its use by cancer patients. Harry Hoxsey ran a cancer clinic from 1936 to 1957 in Dallas, Texas, where he supplied his herbal tonic to patients. In 1963 his long-time nurse, Mildred Nelson, started the Biomedical Center, the first cancer clinic in Tijuana, Mexico, where she continues to administer the Hoxsey tonic to this day. The Hoxsey herbal combination is taken in conjunction with the avoidance of pork, tomato, and vinegar products, under the premise that these foods interfere with the action of the tonic. In clinically-treated cases of skin cancer the Hoxsey tonic is taken in conjunction with topically-applied chemical compounds.

Several of the plants in the tonic have been screened for antitumor activity in various animal tumor systems. While a number of studies were negative, studies of mammary carcinomas transplanted in mice using subdermal injections of extracts of *Stillingia sylvatica*, *Berberis aquifolium*, cascara sagrada, or licorice root reduced the size of the tumors compared to controls in two or more tests by 40-50%, 60-80%, 60-80%, and 50-80%, respectively. As a plant and chemical combination treatment, the Hoxsey tonic has not been tested in controlled studies. Though individual claims of clinical successes and failures have been made, no clinical trials have been reported, nor has any comprehensive independent investigation of the treatment been attempted. Therefore, the Hoxsey tonic has not received federal approval as a treatment for cancer. (See *Unconventional Cancer Treatments*, Chap. 4 "Herbal Treatments," published by the Office of Technology Assessment, Congress of the United States.)

Though similar in content to the Hoxsey tonic, the alterative formula is only intended for cleansing the system by improving elimination of metabolic waste and carries no claims of being a cancer cure. Using it to the exclusion of agents and methods which have been proven effective would be irresponsible and could prove fatal.

Add one of the following formulas if needed.

Immune Support Formula

When the systems of the body need to be cleansed of cellular debris, phagocytosis by white blood cells needs to be encouraged. Echinacea stimulates immune function by activating those cells in the tissues and fluids that eliminate dead or damaged cells and microorganisms. When viral or bacterial lesions or abnormal growths become chronic, cleansing the circulating fluids is an important adjunct in restoring health. The removal of chemical and cellular waste are both necessary to insure a complete resolution of the problem.

Anti-inflammatory Formula

Irritation of tissues in the musculoskeletal system by collected metabolic waste products can induce or aggravate chronic inflammatory conditions of the muscles and joints. Besides alleviating the symptoms of inflammation the processes that initiate the inflammation must be controlled. Stimulating cleansing through the emunctories addresses the possible need for improved removal of endotoxins.

Immune Support Formula

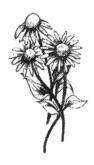

Echinacea, commonly called purple coneflower, has been used in the past as an alterative and antiseptic. Strictly speaking its activity is different from either of these. Although its action was observed to be unique, it was given these labels because it aided in chronic conditions associated with recurrent infections and a "depravation of the body fluids." Recent research and discoveries in immunology has helped us appreciate echinacea's effect on the immune system, such as the enhancement of non-specific resistance. For this purpose echinacea can be taken in a repeating cycle of 3 times per day for 10 days with a 4-day interval in between. Echinacea's high molecular weight polysaccharides (present in the powdered herb or its water extracts but precipitated by concentrated alcohol) have been shown to stimulate white blood cell phagocytic activity. Echinacea extracts also have been shown to stimulate phagocytes in the liver. Other recent discoveries show that the various American species have differing constituents and properties. Thus each species makes its own contribution in optimizing the immune response.

Narrow-leafed echinacea (*Echinacea angustifolia*) root was the first echinacea to be introduced and gain popularity in American medical practice. It was found to increase natural resistance to infections. Its polysaccharide fraction has been shown to have anti-inflammatory activity and immune stimulant proper-

ties. Isobutylamides that stimulate phagocytosis have
been found in the alcoholic extract of this plant. The
root of narrow-leafed echinacea has been shown to
have the highest isobutylamide concentration of all of
the echinacea species tested. It also has small
amounts of antimicrobial polyacetylenes. Its
echinacoside, a caffeic acid glycoside, has shown both
antibacterial and antiviral activity, while cynarin,
another caffeic acid derivative found in the roots, has
demonstrated antitoxin activity in the liver. A major
constituent of the root oil has shown antitumor
activity in cell cultures.

   Tennessee echinacea (*Echinacea tennesseensis*)
root has been shown to have eight isobutylamides
and cynarin in common with the narrow-leafed
echinacea species, but it contains no echinacoside. It
is an endangered species in its wild habitat. In an
effort to preserve the species, only those Tennessee
echinacea plants which have been grown under
cultivation should be used as a source of roots for
herbal remedies.

   Pale echinacea (*Echinacea pallida*) root shares the
antitumor oil constituent and echinacoside with the
narrow-leafed species but contains no cynarin and
very little of the isobutylamides. The roots of pale
echinacea instead have large amounts of phagocyte-
stimulating polyacetylenes which are of a different
type than those found in other species. Both
echinacoside and chicoric acid, a caffeic acid derivative inconsistently present, are antiviral components,
and both are believed to contribute to the immune
stimulation by the alcoholic extract of this plant. The
root of pale echinacea has by far the greatest volatile
oil content of these echinacea species.

   Broad-leafed echinacea (*Echinacea purpurea*) has
become the most cultivated, most studied, and most
used of the various echinacea species. This is largely

because the whole plant (root, leaf, flower, and seed) is used. While the total isobutylamide composition differs between species, the two with strong immunostimulant effects in the root of this broad-leafed species are the same as the major two in narrow-leafed echinacea root. The aerial parts of the plant have a lower concentration of isobutylamides but contain related compounds that are not found in the roots. Polyacetylenes of the same type as in the narrow-leafed species are present though not abundant in broad-leafed echinacea. Chicoric acid is distributed throughout the plant. The high molecular weight polysaccharides are also distributed throughout broad-leafed echinacea and have been shown to activate the large phagocytic white blood cells by promoting the production of tumor necrosis factor, interleukin-1, and interferon-beta$_2$. Injected in mice, these purified high molecular weight polysaccharides increase the growth of phagocytic white blood cells in the spleen and bone marrow, increase their migration into the blood, and protect against lethal infections. Aqueous and alcoholic extracts and the juice from fresh broad-leafed echinacea plants all inhibit viral growth in cell cultures. Extracts of the fresh plants reduced the rate of tissue death in skin flaps. Fresh plant extracts also inhibit the inflammatory swelling due to a foreign substance in test animals. The extract of broad-leafed echinacea helps to prevent the spread of bacteria through tissues by inhibiting the enzyme hyaluronidase which breaks down connective tissue. The stimulation of fibrin-producing cells by its alcoholic extract improves wound healing.

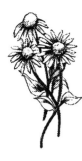

    Echinacea tea made from either the root or root powder contains the high molecular weight polysaccharides. Therefore, the root tea would be good to use as a vehicle for tinctures or formulas used during infections. The root, powder, or alcoholic extract of *E. angustifolia, E. tennesseensis,* or *E. purpurea* should cause a noticeable tingling or numbing sensation on the tongue after a short time. If it does not, then the active isobutylamides are not present. If this is the case the material or extract might either be mislabeled *E. pallida* or some spurious plant.

Add one of the following formulas if needed.

Alterative Formula

In cases of chronic infection where poor elimination of metabolic or environmental toxins burden the immune response, improved waste removal will enhance the cellular defense mechanisms. The immune stimulant alteratives would benefit the process additionally by further stimulating white blood cell reproductive and phagocytic activity.

Antiviral and Antibacterial Formula

Inhibitors of viral growth are not as potent against viruses as antibiotics are against bacteria. Therefore, a concern in viral illness is for optimal immune system function to help contain the virus. Though this is important in acute infections, it is especially true for prolonged cases. Immune stimulation helps prevent complications from secondary bacterial infections.

Cough Relief and Expectorant Formula

Coughs are usually associated with infections. Fighting or "mopping up" an infection always involves the immune system. The more the immune function can be enhanced, the better the defensive response and the quicker the recovery will be.

SUPPORT FOR THE EMUNCTORIES
AND THE IMMUNE SYSTEM

Methods and Agents	Skin	Lungs	Kidneys	Liver	Colon	White Blood Cells	Tissue Phago-cytes
Exercise		•			•		
Sweating	•						
Deep Breathing		•		•			
Fluids			•		•		
Fiber					•		
Fasting			•	•	•		
Colonics				•	•		
Hydrotherapy	•		•	•		•	•
Massage	•					•	•
Vitamin C				•		•	•
Beta-Carotene		•				•	•
Zinc						•	•
Potassium Iodide		•					
Herbs							
Red Clover		•		•		•	
Burdock	•		•		•	•	
Licorice					•	•	
Oregon Grape	•		•	•	•	•	
Buckthorn					•		
Cascara Sagrada				•	•		
Prickly Ash	•		•				
Queen's Root		•					
Echinacea				•		•	•
Prevention							
Avoid Allergens	•	•			•	•	•
Washing	•						
Waste Disposal				•			
Clean Air		•		•			
Organic Food			•	•			
Cooking					•		

II

NUTRITION & DIGESTION

Dietary Content And Habits

Selecting the appropriate food and drink, finding a comfortable setting in which to eat, and taking the necessary time to enjoy the experience allows the digestive system to extract the most nutrition from the food.

The appetite, or desire for food, is influenced by many things. Infancy experiences of satisfaction are intimately related to the act of eating. Besides just satisfying hunger and thirst, diets are influenced by enjoyment from pleasurable flavors, associations of food with memorable events, personal appearance, guilt, other's expectations, convenience, availability, cost, and knowledge of nutrition. Dietary preferences are determined by these and other factors. Sometimes poor food choices are made through habit or are due to inner compulsions that are difficult to resist. The ease of using nutritionally-depleted processed foods makes them attractive to a cook who is fatigued. Just as nutritional information is sought, attempts to control the appetites through different techniques are made. Yet instead of developing assurance, controversies over the best forms, combinations, and amounts of nutrients and ways of preparing food often create more confusion.

Apart from individual food sensitivities, the basis for a wholesome diet remains simple. **Foods are most beneficial when they are grown organically, prepared fresh, eaten in moderation according to need, and enjoyed.** The major source of calories to supply steady energy should be complex carbohydrates obtained from whole grains and their products. These also provide necessary fiber in the diet. Sources of protein are needed in smaller amounts for growth and repair. These include nuts, legumes, and good quality dairy and/or meat products. With the exception of fish the consumption of animal products and nuts should be limited due to their fat content. Small amounts of unsaturated (liquid) vegetable oils provide essential fatty acids for healthy metabolism. Fresh and cooked vegetables provide important sources of starch, soluble fiber, vitamins, minerals, flavonoids, and other micronutrients for meals. Rather than starches, fruits contain simple sugars that supply rapid energy and so should be eaten fresh apart from other foods that require more digestion. They are excellent sources of the other factors found in vegetables. **Adequate fluid intake, especially pure water, is essential but should be supplied mostly between meals.** Small quantities of warm, aromatic herbal teas taken with meals can enhance digestion.

Along with these guidelines for good eating, certain other choices are important to avoid dietary health problems. Digestion is made simpler if carbo-hydrates and proteins are not eaten at the same meal. Fried food should be kept to a minimum. Concen-trated sweets are best taken in small amounts on special occasions or for some people not used at all. Salt should be used in moderation and many other food additives should be avoided entirely. **Food allergies involving commonly consumed foods are**

believed to contribute to a significant portion of chronic health problems. Common allergens are found in cow's milk, eggs, wheat, corn, and oranges or their byproducts. Many allergies seem to arise from introducing the food too early in infancy such as giving cow's milk to babies before they are one year old.

It is often said, "You are what you eat," but the truth is that we can be malnourished even when our diet is optimal. **If our dietary habits are inappropriate, our digestion will suffer and what we absorb and assimilate could be deficient.** While a small drink of cool water before a meal can stimulate our stomach and prepare it for food, large quantities of iced drinks during or after a meal suppresses and dilutes digestive secretions. We live in a fast-paced society where there is an emphasis on production and a premium on time. Meals are often eaten in a rush or under stressful conditions such as at a working environment or in traffic. Under these circumstances the full flavor of food cannot be enjoyed, nor can it be adequately mixed with digestive fluids. Digestion begins in the mouth when chewing mixes the food with saliva which breaks down carbohydrates. When in a hurry to finish, diners do not chew long or well enough.

The autonomic nervous system (regulates organ function unconsciously through adrenergic and cholinergic nerves) is strongly influenced by our attitudes and surroundings. **Digestion is affected by the mental and physical environment in which we eat.** Hurried activity combined with stress from the surroundings causes the adrenergic nerves (control fright, flight, or fight response to adrenaline) to take over. This sends more blood to the muscles and brain and shuts down the digestion. Whatever the type of job and its stresses, working after a meal makes digestion difficult. A peaceful atmosphere helps put the cholinergic nerves (produce relaxation response to acetylcholine) in control. This moves the blood more to the gastrointestinal tract as the activity of digestive organs increases. A period of rest after a meal, the well-known siesta of many foreign lands, optimizes digestion. The ideal circumstances are improbable in our society. When the proper conditions are not possible due to occupational demands, it is better to eat only as necessary. Foods requiring little digestion like soups, salads, or fruit should be consumed at these times. In some situations it may even be best to skip a meal, especially if loss of appetite, an upset stomach, or nausea are already present.

Stomach And Gall Bladder

The absorption of nutrients requires the adequate breakdown of whole foods. This digestive process is a series of steps that involve secretions from several different organs. The optimal function of each one is necessary to obtain the best digestion and prevent abdominal discomfort. If dyspepsia does occur, irritation and spasms can be relieved.

Although we may be careful about what and how we eat, poor digestive function or dietary intolerances may still interfere with our receiving the best nourishment possible. Digestion is completed in the small intestine where pancreatic enzymes are released that break down carbohydrates, proteins, and fats. **Just as digestion of carbohydrates begins in the mouth, so the digestion of protein starts in the stomach and fat breakdown is initiated by the gall bladder emptying into the small intestine.** Insufficient protein digestion may be caused by a lack of secretion of gastric (stom-

ach) acid. Incomplete breakdown of protein can lead
to absorption of large molecules that trigger allergic
reactions to food. Diminished bile from the gall
bladder results in poorly emulsified oils and reduced
digestion and absorption of essential fatty acids.

Deficient digestion is usually chronic. Diminished function frequently develops in old age or after
mental/emotional stress (anxiety). It is often associated with anorexia (loss of appetite). Poor digestion
also occurs after the anorexia of acute fevers or
inflammatory diseases. These conditions require
tonics (agents that restore activity) to support digestion. Protecting the sensitive lining of the gut is
another concern in the process of increasing stomach
acid and gall bladder secretions. **Some individuals
react to particular foods, food additives, contaminants, or drugs to which they are sensitive.** These
reactions may be in the form of gastrointestinal
allergies, essential intolerances, excessive intake of a
particular substance, or as a result of inappropriate
combinations. Besides avoiding the causes these cases
can be aided by neutralizing irritations and improving digestive activity, as well as by using carminatives
(agents that relax intestinal spasms).

**Both inadequate breakdown of food and reac-
tions to food can cause indigestion.** The uncomfortable symptoms of functional dyspepsia can arise
during or after a meal. They include nausea, a heavy
sensation in the stomach, heartburn, stomachache,
cramping, bloating, "rumbling," or gas. Food that is
not adequately digested and absorbed provides an
ideal medium for bacterial fermentation in the gut.
This can produce some of the symptoms after meals.
Vomiting or diarrhea can occur in severe reactions or
in cases where the system is incapable of digestion.
X-ray studies are necessary to determine whether

there is any ulceration or malignancy associated with these symptoms. X-ray diagnosis is essential if there is any evidence of bleeding (such as bloody or "coffee ground" vomit or black, tarry stools). Once the problem has been accurately identified, supportive measures can be used and eating habits adjusted to overcome these problems. **If it is necessary to improve secretions from the stomach or gall bladder on a regular basis, certain tonic herbs can assist. When aggravating items are consumed and acute relief is needed, carminative herbs are indicated.**

Bitter Digestive Tonic Formula

Bitter tonics have been used for generations as a means of increasing digestive efficiency. The fact that bitter is one of the four primary tastes suggests it has a functional significance. Plant alkaloids are bitter and some can be toxic in overdose. Therefore, this tasting ability is probably a physiological means to avoid poisonings. The typical digestive tract response to most toxic plants is hyperstimulation. This culminates in vomiting and diarrhea to expel the material. Small doses of the tonic bitters provide a lesser degree of stimulation. The digestive activity is safely heightened without purging. Cases of functional dyspepsia associated with emotional and/or autonomic imbalance have been known to benefit from this influence. Specific indications for the use of bitters include chronic gastritis with low acid output and reduced gall bladder secretion. Tonic bitters also act as an appetite stimulant in cases where the desire for food has been lost. This activity is aided by aromatics and flavoring agents that help to increase secretions of the alimentary mucosa. Soothing demulcents help to prevent irritation to the stomach lining.

Gentian (*Gentiana lutea*) root acts both as a stomachic to increase stomach acid production and as a choleretic to stimulate the secretion of bile. It contains a number of bitter secoiridoid glycosides common to its genus and is the most frequently used bitter tonic herb. Gentian stimulates stomach motility through the cholinergic nerves, but it does not speed stomach emptying. Though gentian inhibits the sensations of fullness, it does not increase the rate of weight gain during growth. Several of the glycosides in gentian root have shown anti-inflammatory activity and help prevent gastric ulcer formation. **However, gentian should not be used in acute gastric inflammation or ulceration due to hyperacidity of the stomach because of its powerful stomachic properties.**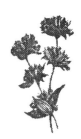

Goldenseal (*Hydrastis canadensis*) is another bitter root used as a stomachic tonic. It is taken especially for chronic inflammation of the stomach where there is excessive mucus production. Goldenseal is even more effective than gentian at stimulating stomach acid secretion. It contains several alkaloids of which berberine is foremost. Berberine increases intestinal tone. Goldenseal's effects may be mainly due to berberine's activity that inhibits the enzymatic breakdown of the cholinergic neurotransmitter. Berberine greatly increases bile secretion for one and a half hours after it is taken. Its regular use relieved the symptoms of patients with chronic gall bladder inflammation and led to an increased concentration of their bile. Berberine's antimicrobial activity helps to reduce fermentation in the intestines along with the associated symptoms.

Angelica (*Angelica archangelica*, also called *A. officinalis*) root is not only a bitter stomachic and appetite stimulant. It also has a carminative action that relieves gas and intestinal spasms. The latter effects are due to its aromatic oils which are mostly terpene alcohols. These aromatics have been used to flavor several well-known herbal liqueurs. Its bitter components are furanocoumarins. They act by blocking calcium uptake in gland cells.

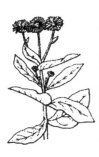

Elecampane (*Inula helenium*) root has been used both as an aromatic bitter stomachic and as a chola-gogue to stimulate bile flow. Its activity is attributed to helenin, a volatile oil mixture made up mostly of alantolactone. Elecampane's effectiveness for ulcers is probably due to helenin's hemostatic properties. Helenin has been shown to decrease bleeding time and blood loss.

Fennel (*Foeniculum vulgare*) seeds have demon-strated an ability to stimulate stomach and small intestine motility. This action is associated with the cholinergic neurotransmitter and its precursor which are found in roasted fennel seeds. Fennel seed alco-holic extract was shown to be antispasmodic in contractions of the small intestine caused by hista-mine. This action is at least partially due to fennel's aromatic oil which consists of mostly anethole. This oil is often used for its licorice-like flavor. It acts as a carminative for intestinal cramps. Anethole also has been shown to increase bile flow.

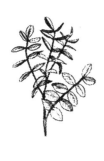

Licorice (*Glycyrrhiza glabra*) root is a soothing demulcent with a sweet flavor. It helps mask the intense bitterness of the tonic herbs. Licorice has been used for the prevention and treatment of peptic ulcers. Carbenoxolone, a synthetic drug derived from glycyrrhetic acid in licorice, stimulates mucus secretion of stomach cells. It has been used success-fully to treat ulcers. However, problems of develop-ing low potassium and high blood pressure occurred in some individuals (about 20%) after prolonged carbenoxolone use. To avoid such problems the regular use of plain licorice tea is also inadvisable. A deglycyrrhizinated licorice extract was developed and found to be effective without noticeable side effects. Problems from regular use of whole licorice root can be prevented by keeping the dosage low as part of a combination and resting periodically from its use. It is advisable to supplement potassium and/or methionine. **Those with high blood pressure or heart failure should avoid its long-term use at high doses.**

To aid in digestion the tonic should be taken in a little water one half hour before meals. It needs to be used persistently to improve and maintain the digestive response. The licorice helps insure tolerance to both the taste and the stomachic effects. Otherwise, gastric irritation or nausea might occur if pure bitters were taken on an empty stomach. This formula is not intended for peptic ulcers or acute inflammation of the stomach. Its effect of increasing the acid in the stomach could aggravate the ulcers and inflammation.

Add the following formula if needed.

Soothing Sleep and Sedative Formula

When stress or anxiety diminish digestive activity, a preparation that reduces mental tension and improves relaxation can help to improve digestion. The use of a small amount of this combination prior to a meal can set the tone for a pleasant, nourishing experience.

Carminative Antacid and Flavoring Formula

Dyspepsia symptoms after meals sometimes indicate irritation of the digestive apparatus. In these acute cases it may be necessary to use a combination that provides symptomatic relief while improving digestion in the intestines. Carminative herbs relax intestinal spasms and ease discomfort. Excessive acidity is a common cause of burning pain that requires intervention. The antacid in the formula neutralizes acidity. When acid is not adequately neutralized, the development of aggravation of peptic ulcers is a possibility. In addition, pancreatic digestive enzymes released in the small intestine are not effective in acid. Reduced enzyme activity can lead to bloating, gas pains, or diarrhea, due in part to bacterial fermentation of undigested food in the intestinal tract. Cholagogue herbs in the following formula stimulate bile release from the gall bladder which enhances digestion after consumption of rich foods.

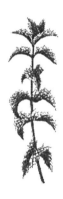

Peppermint (Mentha piperita) oil has an obvious presence in this formula due to its familiar fragrance and taste. The mild anesthetic property of menthol, the major terpene component in the oil, helps to ease discomfort by allaying uncomfortable sensations such as nausea. Menthol also acts as a stomachic by increasing stomach muscular activity. Peppermint extract, oil, and menthol all reduce spastic activity in the intestine that is caused by histamine and cholinergic stimuli. Peppermint oil also helps relax the sphincter muscles of the digestive tract to allow easier passage of gases. It has an inhibitory effect on bacterial fermentation due to the mildly antiseptic activity of the aromatic oil and the menthol. Both menthol and another aromatic component, menthone, have choleretic activity that increases bile flow for hours after being taken orally.

Cinnamon (Cinnamomum cassia) bark also has carminative properties that helps relax intestinal contractions. Studied as a major component in a combination of herbs with digestive enzymes or antacids, it helped inhibit ulcer development from aspirin use. Cinnamon does not affect stomach

movement. A water extract of cinnamon showed
potent anti-complement activity that reduced the
allergic response. This extract contained four types
of diterpenes, mostly cinncassiols. The aromatic oil
of cinnamon and its main component,
cinnamaldehyde, are both antibacterial.

Goldenseal (*Hydrastis canadensis*) root is a
berberine-containing tonic that is traditionally used
for ulcers. Berberine stimulates bile secretion. It is
especially helpful in cases of chronic inflammation of
the gall bladder. Berberine's antimicrobial activity
helps to reduce gas production caused by fermentation of undigested foods. It also inhibits the secretory effects of the intestinal toxins that certain bacteria produce. Its ability to reduce diarrhea secretions
helps to control excessive fluid loss from physiologic
stimulants or food poisoning. Diarrhea and amebic
dysentery may be offset by sufficient doses of berberine even in children.

Rhubarb (*Rheum spp.*) root is usually considered
a laxative because of its anthroquinone derivatives.
However, the highest concentration, most potent
anthroquinones, and strongest laxative effect are
found only in the roots of Chinese rhubarb species
(*R. palmatum* or *R. officinale*). In small amounts
rhubarb root acts as an appetite stimulant and digestive tonic that enhances liver and gall bladder activity.
It is astringent because of its tannin content. The
tannin components also act to protect the liver cell
membranes from peroxidation damage.

Potassium bicarbonate is an antacid compound
that neutralizes and alleviates acid indigestion. It
affords relief for heartburn from stomach contents
which escape back up into the esophagus and cause
irritation. In this combination it provides another
function beyond the stomach. It neutralizes the acid

and enzymes from the stomach when they pass into the small intestine and helps to prevent ulceration there. Also, the pancreatic digestive enzymes that mix with the food in the small intestine require a neutral or alkaline medium to be effective. The bicarbonate helps both to protect the gut and aid in digestion when used a short while after a meal. Potassium is used instead of sodium because of physiological advantages unrelated to digestion.

Vegetable glycerin is an important component in this formula. It acts as a solvent and preservative in combination with distilled water and alcohol. Glycerin provides a sweet-tasting component without the use of sugar. It is soothing to the membrane lining of the gut. Since its use dilutes the mixture the dosage for this formula is greater than for others. Doses are two teaspoonsful taken every one to four hours as needed. A child's dose is about one fourth this amount. Children favor this remedy because of its pleasant taste.

This combination was an improvement made by the renowned Lloyd Brothers Pharmacists on a widely popular neutralizing cordial. It was originally used by eclectic medical doctors as both an agent for gastrointestinal disorders and as a vehicle to flavor bitter or distasteful remedies. In some cases herbal remedies taken between meals can produce symptoms of nausea because of the taste of the herbs or their local action in the stomach. As a flavoring vehicle the carminative antacid combination prevents stomach upset caused by other medicines.

Add one of the following formulas if needed.

Anthelmintic Formula

The bitterness of some components used against worms sometimes makes it necessary to use a flavorful vehicle for oral consumption, especially for children. The aromatics of cinnamon and peppermint in both of these combinations helps ease the bitter effect on the stomach and prevent the nausea that can occur when it is used between meals. The additional peppermint, cinnamon and goldenseal in the flavoring vehicle will also aid the antiparasite activity of the Anthelmintic Formula.

Liver Tonic Formula

In cases with both excessive stomach acid and an intolerance to oily foods, biliary effects can be enhanced by using other herbs that stimulate bile secretions by the liver. This is an especially useful addition when the gall bladder, which only concentrates the bile and controls its release after meals, contains stones or has been surgically removed. The tonic herbs also are helpful for protecting the liver from damage from alcohol or drugs. The bitter flavor of the liver tonic will sometimes require a flavorful vehicle to make it more tolerable.

Antiseptic Formula

The flavor of the antiseptic formula is somewhat bitter when used internally. Together these formulas can better relieve the digestive discomfort and intestinal gas caused by bacterial fermentation. They can also help control the symptoms of vomiting and diarrhea from acute gastrointestinal infections.

OPTIMIZING NOURISHMENT AND
REDUCING DISCOMFORT FROM FOOD

SELECTING FOODS FOR GREATEST BENEFITS

Qualities	Menu	Avoid	Don't Eat When
Nutritious	Nuts	Refined Foods	Anxious or Upset
Organic	Beans	Processed foods	Actively Working
Flavorful	Dairy	Fried Foods	In a Hurry
Fresh	Fish or Meat	Fruit with Meals	In Acute Pain
Affordable	Vegetables	Sweets	Stomach Is Upset
	Fresh Fruit	Additives	Appetite
	Unsaturated	Intolerances	Temporarily Lost
	Oils	Combining	Nauseous
	Whole Grain	Incompatibles	
	Products	**Excessive:**	
	Herb Teas	Salt	
	Water	Oils & Fats	
		Fluids with Meals	
		Protein with Meals	

ENHANCING DIGESTION   RELIEVING INDIGESTION

Utilize	Avoid	Utilize	Avoid
Quiet	Stress	Rest	Stress
Relaxation	Rushing	Antacids	Eating
Chewing	Noise	**Demulcents:**	Purgatives
Savoring	Confusion	Licorice	
Aromatics:	Iced drinks	Glycerin	
Fennel	Overindulgence	**Cholagogues:**	
Bitters:		Goldenseal	
Gentian		Rhubarb Root	
Angelica		**Carminatives:**	
Goldenseal		Peppermint	
Elecampane		Cinnamon	

III

PROTECTION & ELIMINATION

Liver And Colon

The proper function of the liver is essential to protect the body from toxic chemicals, but the liver itself is susceptible to damage and sometimes needs protection. Dietary fiber from whole foods is a helpful means of promoting elimination of toxins through the colon. When parasites inhabit the intestinal tract their elimination requires more potent agents.

The liver processes toxins including both metabolic waste products that are formed within the body and poisons that are absorbed from outside the body. The liver metabolizes solvents used in industry and household cleansing, chemicals used in raising crops and livestock, food additives, pollutants in the air and water, and prescription medicines and recreational drugs such as alcohol. These can become so concentrated that they destroy normal liver function. They can even cause fatal poisoning.

It is important to avoid exposure to environmental toxins whenever possible. It is also desirable to promote their rapid elimination. Sometimes they pass from the body intact without being chemically changed. Frequently, however, chemicals absorbed into the blood are altered by cells in the liver or chemically bound as a way to protect the system. When the liver works effectively the processed toxins can be released back into the blood for excretion from the lungs if they are gaseous or through the kidneys if they are water soluble. They can also be secreted with the bile into the gall bladder to be excreted through the intestines. **If the liver is exposed to high levels of toxins suddenly or to low levels of poisons on a regular basis, it can become inflamed and no longer function efficiently.** The liver's integrity is necessary for health since it contributes in many ways to normal biological activity. Some of its vital functions include providing nutrient storage and conversions and producing blood clotting factors. **Certain herbs can help protect the liver from damage due to chemical exposure and support its functions.**

Fiber provided by whole foods in the diet is beneficial for optimal liver function. The liver converts cholesterol into bile salts. These salts are secreted with the bile which is stored and concentrated in the gall bladder. Bile is released into the intestines after a meal to emulsify the fats in food. Some of the bile salts and other compounds in the bile are bound to the water-soluble, noncellulose plant fiber and eliminated through the colon. These bile salts that are not reabsorbed act on the colon in a laxative manner. The soluble fiber also prevents atrophy of the colon lining. Some of the water-soluble fiber is broken down by bacteria to short chain fatty acids, providing fuel for the cells lining the colon. This fiber breakdown produces an acid bowel environment which promotes the growth of beneficial bacteria and inhibits growth of harmful microorganisms. Much of the fiber in food from plants is cellulose which cannot be digested. Along with water and bacteria the cellulose provides much of the bulk of fecal waste that is to be eliminated.

By holding biliary products in the bowel, fiber stimulates the colon and aids in elimination of toxins and cholesterol products. It also acts as a stimulus to colon muscles for evacuation by absorbing water and providing bulk. More rapid movement of waste through the bowel reduces the reabsorption of fecal compounds. In addition, the protective effect of high fiber diets against the development of colon cancer may be due in part to this rapid transit time. Other factors also are involved in reducing bowel cancer risk with fiber. Fecal toxin concentration is diluted, and bacterial conversion of precursors to cancer-causing agents is reduced. The properties of fiber make it a necessary element in the diet. Fiber sources cannot be replaced simply by reliance on laxatives or enemas to promote elimination.

In contrast to modern concerns about toxin exposure an old problem involving elimination from the colon is the expulsion of parasites. These enter the body, usually with food, and proliferate in the bowels. In primitive cultures a periodic ritual cleansing with cathartic herbs was used to purge the system of worms associated with unhygienic lifestyles and dietary practices. Modern food handling and treatment techniques have eliminated much of the potential for infestation. Untold opportunities for the acquisition of various worms are still provided by the consumption of under-cooked meat or fish or contact with animal waste (usually by children, particularly if barefoot). Once established, worms are spread to others through poor hygiene. They may cause no symptoms, or they may produce respiratory effects or abdominal pain and chronic bowel complaints. They sometimes make their appearance in the stools. In the case of common pinworms they congregate outside to lay eggs at night which causes anal itching.

These insidious invaders rob the host by consuming nutrients which results in weight loss and deficiencies. Active efforts are required for their removal. Worms are more readily dispatched when deprived of protein by fasting. Eating raw pineapple or figs that contain proteolytic enzymes works in conjunction with fasting as a vermicide by helping to dissolve the surface of roundworms. Large quantities of pumpkin seeds contain a safe vermifugal substance that paralyzes tapeworms. Irritating foods also reduce their attachment to the intestinal wall. **In the case of worm infestation a combination of laxatives and herbs toxic to the worms is useful to promote their evacuation.**

Liver Tonic Formula

A major concern in supporting the metabolic functions of the liver is protecting it against damage from poisonous substances and viral infections. The best means of protecting it from harmful substances is by avoiding exposure to toxins and eliminating their consumption. Another way is by supplementing antioxidants. Using herbal compounds and extracts to prevent liver damage and aid recovery has produced dramatic results in laboratory tests that are confirmed by clinical trials. Choleretic herbs, commonly called liver tonics, act on the liver to produce more bile and improve the rate of clearing the biliary products from this organ. This increased bile output contributes to their reputation as mild laxatives. Some choleretics are reputed to reduce the congestion in the liver and spleen when they are enlarged from infections.

Milk thistle (*Silybum marianum*, formerly called *Carduus marianus*) seeds have been used both for

liver troubles and associated enlargement of the
spleen. They contain a group of flavonolignans
known collectively as silymarin, the major component of which is silybin. Silybin is remarkable for its
protection against poisoning by the deathcap toad-
stool, and silymarin is also curative for the damage
from the components of this fungus. Silymarin is
nontoxic and prevents or reduces liver toxicity caused
by carbon tetrachloride, thioacetamide, galac-
tosamine, and thallium Silybin has these effects in
cases of halothane anesthesia and acetaminophen
overdose. Silymarin protects liver cells from viral
damage and speeds the rate of liver regeneration. It
produced positive results in several clinical studies on
chronic hepatitis. Silymarin protects the liver from
acute high levels of ethanol, helps normalize cellular
changes in mild acute and subacute alcohol damage,
and reduces mortality from alcoholic cirrhosis. It
also helps prevent drug metabolism disorders in cases
where there is pre-existing liver damage or cirrhosis.

Dandelion (*Taraxacum officinale*) root is a
stimulant for bile secretions. As a choleretic it has
been used both as a means of removing toxins from
the system and as a tonic to improve digestion.
Applications of dandelion root have included all
varieties of liver problems. It contains the triterpene
alcohols taraxerol and taraxasterol which are common to other bitter liver tonics, also. Sitosterol is an
important component of both roots and leaves which
produces anti-inflammatory effects when given
orally. Dandelion roots and leaves are diuretics with
the leaves being the more potent. They have demonstrated the ability to help flush salts and water weight
from the system.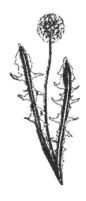

Oregon grape (*Berberis aquifolium,* also called
Mahonia aquifolium) root contains berberine and is

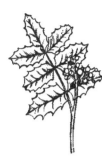

considered a tonic for the liver and gastrointestinal tract. It mildly stimulates stomach acid secretion and has some laxative effect, possibly due to berberine's enhancement of bile flow. The alkaloidal components berberine, oxyacanthine, and berbamine all are potent stimulants of biliary secretion. Both berberine and jatrorrhizine, another alkaloid component, showed anti-inflammatory activity and improved recovery from liver damage caused by thioacetamide. Patients with toxic hepatitis due to industrial poisons showed improvement in their condition after taking berberine.

The most common application of **red root** (*Ceanothus americanus*) for problems of the liver is for cases where it is enlarged and painful due to inflammation. In cases of infections where there is also enlargement of the spleen, it has been used to reduce congestion of both these organs. It contains the peptide alkaloids ceanothine-B, -C, -D, and -E and ceanothamine-A and -B. Four dicarboxylic and two phosphoric acids from red root reduce the time it takes for blood to clot due to their effect on blood calcium. The cascade of clotting factors formed by the liver are activated by calcium in the blood.

This combination should be taken three times each day. In cases where there is a need for greater secretion of bile to aid digestion, such as after gall bladder removal or when the gall bladder volume is reduced by stones, it should be used after meals. It will be particularly beneficial for discomfort from eating foods that are too high in fat.

Add one of the following formulas if needed.

Carminative Antacid and Flavoring Formula

The bitter taste of some liver tonic herbs makes certain individuals unwilling to use them. By taking these bitters with a sweet, pleasant flavoring agent that also settles the stomach, the beneficial effects can be gained without undergoing a distasteful experience.

Venous Tonic Formula

In attempting to resolve problems of venous bulging it is necessary to correct the cause. The development of protruding internal hemorrhoids is sometimes caused by congestion of the liver and associated constipation which produces a back-pressure in the veins around the anus. The liver tonics, in helping to resolve the congestion and constipation, reduce the pressure that causes these veins to bulge.

Premenstrual Ease Formula

The involvement of the liver in estrogen metabolism is a consideration in conditions having high estrogen levels. Improving the conversion of circulating estrogens to less active forms can be an effective part of controlling premenstrual problems. Addressing this association may be the first and most important aspect of regaining hormonal balance and relieving symptoms.

Anthelmintic Formula

The various anthelmintic (anti-worm) herbs affect different parasitic worms. Combining anthelmintics that promote their expulsion allows a broad application for worm infestations. While the vermicides actually kill the worms, vermifuges weaken or immobilize them so that they can be removed by purging. After symptoms have subsided stool analysis is used to determine that no worms or their eggs still remain. Otherwise, the infestation may become re-established. In cases where parasites have travelled from the intestines and invaded other organs or tissues, further medical intervention is required.

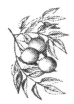

The fresh, green hulls of the **black walnut** (*Juglans nigra*) are used because they contain juglone and related compounds that are not found in the dry, blackened hulls. The juice from these hulls has been used in cases of worms and locally for certain skin diseases. Juglone acts as a depressant for fish and the smooth muscle of the intestines. This correlates with the vermifuge action required to weaken and remove worms. Juglans species with juglone have been used as anthelmintics for tapeworms, pinworms, and threadworms. Juglone is effective for local infections because of its antifungal activity, the inhibition of Staph. and Candida, and blocking enzymes necessary for replication of certain viruses.

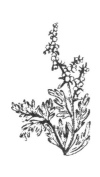

Wormwood (*Artemisia absinthium*) takes its name from a long tradition of use as a vermicide against ascarides (roundworms) and tapeworms. The leaves of this herbaceous (not woody) plant are extremely bitter, but the activity is due mostly to the aromatic oil they contain. They have also been used as a stomachic, as a cholagogue, and as a carminative for digestive complaints. The major component in this oil is thujone, but pinene and cineole are other important constituents. These three compounds all show anthelmintic activity against ascarides.

Thyme (*Thymus vulgaris*) leaves are also used as an anthelmintic and as a carminative for digestive complaints. They are valued because of their aromatic oil which contains varying amounts of thymol, carvacrol, geraniol, and cineole. Thymol is the major constituent that is responsible for its vermicidal effects on ascarides, pinworms, and especially hookworms, but carvacrol, geraniol, and cineole are likewise effective for ascarides. Flavonoids in thyme, as well as thymol and carvacrol, relieve spasms in the intestines.

Quassia (*Picrasma excelsa*) wood is another anthelmintic plant with a strong bitter taste. In this case the bitterness is due to quassinoids and alkaloids. It is taken internally or used in an enema to kill pinworms. It is also taken orally as a vermifuge for threadworms, but is especially indicated for ascarides.

Cinnamon (*Cinnamomum cassia*) bark with its aromatic cinnamaldehyde component is carminative, as well as being anthelmintic against ascarides and pinworms.

Peppermint (*Mentha piperita*) oil constituents menthol and menthone show vermicidal activity against ascarides. The oil is also carminative, relaxing bowel spasms because of the high menthol content.

Cascara sagrada (*Rhamnus purshiana*) aged bark is useful in this combination to cause evacuation of the bowels after the parasites have been immobilized or killed. Its cascaroside anthroquinones stimulate the rhythmic muscular contractions of the intestines and keep sufficient fluid in the gut to expel bowel contents easily.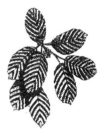

A typical adult dose would be 1/4 - 1 teaspoon taken 1 -3 times daily. It is taken in the morning after fasting since the previous evening's supper. It may then be repeated in the afternoon between meals, and taken again at bedtime. After several days of using this remedy the final dose can be taken in the morning and followed after several hours by Epsom salts mixed with iced orange juice as a purgative.

Add the following formula if needed.

Carminative Antacid and Flavoring Formula

The pleasant flavor and soothing effects on the stomach and intestinal tract help this combination make the use of bitter anthelmintic and laxative herbs much easier to tolerate at effective dosage levels. The additional peppermint and cinnamon aromatic oils also favor the antihelmintic effect.

CLEANSING OF THE COLON AND LIVER

LIVER HEALTH

Systemic and Liver Toxins	Provides Liver Protection	Enhances Toxin Excretion
Solvents	Water-soluble Fiber	Water-soluble Fiber
Pesticides	Antioxidants	**Choleretics:**
Food Additives	Milk Thistle	Dandelion Root
Environmental Pollutants	Oregon Grape	Oregon Grape
Drugs	Red Root	
Alcohol		
Viral Infections		

COLON EVACUATION

Normal Bowel Contents	Colon Irritants	Enhances Colon Emptying	Alleviates Bowel Cramps	Expels Worms
Fiber	Bacterial Products	Fiber	Wormwood	Cathartics
Bile Salts	Parasites	Bile Salts	Thyme	Fasting
Undigested Food	Bile Salts	Water	Cinnamon	Pineapple
Bacteria	Casgada Sagrada	Enemas	Peppermint	Figs
Water		**Laxatives:**		Pumpkin Seeds
		Casgada Sagrada		Black Walnut Husk
		Epsom Salts		Wormwood
				Thyme
				Quassia
				Cinnamon
				Peppermint

Kidneys And Bladder

Filtering the blood through the kidneys removes most of its soluble waste particles. Sufficient fluid intake provides the means to avoid concentrated urine. Urine retention and infection of the bladder should be prevented when possible or treated early to avoid kidney involvement.

Water-soluble waste products (such as urea from the ammonia formed during protein degradation) are released by the liver into the circulation to join other cellular waste and nutrients in the blood plasma. **The function of the kidneys is to filter certain soluble components out of the blood and maintain the fluid balance in the body.** It does so by allowing compounds in the blood that are smaller than proteins to pass into its tubules. Some are actively reabsorbed from the filtrate back into the blood such as glucose, amino acids, some vitamins, calcium, magnesium, and sodium. Potassium and urates are actively secreted into the filtrate. Some water passes back out, but other substances cannot easily pass back through the membrane. This is the case with urea, urates, nitrates, sulfates, and phosphates. **These substances together with the water lost are excreted as urine.** High concentrations of certain compounds, too much or too little acid in the urine, and urine retention help cause the formation of gravel from crystals in the kidneys. The fluid balance and active reabsorption is under hormonal control. However, urinary output is also influenced by blood flow to the kidneys, the concentration of protein in the blood, blood pressure, and osmotic diuretics. **Excretion of waste in the urine can be promoted by generous consumption of pure water.**

The urine that is formed is collected in the bladder. Here it is held until the amount is sufficient to stretch the bladder muscle and stimulate contraction and voiding. **When there is prolonged retention of the urine (due to social or occupational demands or anatomical conditions), the bladder becomes more vulnerable and the opportunity for both the formation of gravel and bacterial growth is enhanced.** Irritation occurring from gravel in the urine can increase susceptibility to infection. There is an increased risk of bladder infection in women due to the its close proximity to a bacteria-rich exterior, especially when the bladder is full and exposed to trauma during sexual intercourse. The presence of sugar in the urine provides food for microorganisms and further promotes their growth. Infections can cause symptoms such as a sense of urgency to urinate and frequent, burning, or painful urination. (Blood in the urine, especially if there are no other accompanying symptoms, signals an immediate need for a medical examination.) The discomfort during urination is what usually alerts a person to the need for intervention.

The main danger of bladder infections is the risk of their spreading to the kidneys. Involvement of these vital organs, which do not have the high concentration of immune system cells that protect the lungs and liver, can cause severe illness. Symptoms of kidney infections include fever, pain in the lower back, and general toxicity and indicate a serious medical condition. **To prevent kidney involvement it is important to control infections of the bladder and not to allow them to progress beyond the earliest symptoms.** Avoiding the predisposing factors for these infections is a helpful means of control. Regular or periodic consumption of cranberry products is a popular and effective means of preventing bladder infections for those who are most susceptible such as the elderly or others in nursing homes.

Diuretic and Urinary Antiseptic Formula

This combination unites herbs that affect the kidneys and bladder in different ways. Some of the herbs help increase urine output and flush the urinary tract, while others reduce symptoms of irritation by their soothing properties. Certain herbs contain antimicrobial constituents that inhibit bacterial growth by their antiseptic effect and reduce bacterial adherence. One helps increase the immune response. The intended effects are to dilute the urine, make it less favorable for gravel formation and bacterial growth, overcome discomforts associated with lower urinary tract inflammation, and prevent the spread of bacteria to the kidneys.

Uva ursi (*Arctostaphylos uva-ursi*) leaves are used for a variety of bladder problems. These relieve irritation and bleeding caused by gravel in the kid-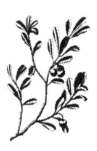neys and help prevent urate crystal accumulation. Uva ursi extract is especially important as a urinary antiseptic against E. coli and Proteus bacteria because of the high arbutin content of the leaves. The glyco-side arbutin is broken down to hydroquinone espe-cially in alkaline urine where it acts as a disinfectant. **Excessive hydroquinone can irritate the liver.** Uva ursi also contains ursolic acid which is antiseptic for both gram-positive and gram-negative bacteria and yeasts. Uva ursi and its arbutin and ursolic acid are also anti-inflammatory. Other phenolic and fla-vonoid constituents including oleanolic acid, gallic acid, and quercetin were shown to contribute to the antimicrobial and anti-inflammatory effects as well. **The tannins in uva ursi can upset the stomach in large amounts.**

Horsetail (*Equisetum arvense*) stems have a

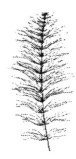

diuretic activity that increases the flow of urine. This helps to flush the crystalline wastes from the tract before they can coalesce to form gravel. The active components, most likely saponins, are present in alcoholic extracts. Isoquercitrin is its major flavonoid. Besides reducing the irritation, horsetail is used as a hemostatic agent to stop bleeding due to gravel or infections.

The flowers of **goldenrod** (*Solidago canadensis*) have similar constituents and activity to European goldenrod but are more potent as diuretics. By its action on the kidneys goldenrod lowers the urea nitrogen level in the blood. It has several flavonoid glycosides but quercitrin is seen as the most important for reducing bleeding due to kidney inflammation. Its eleven saponins, including the sapogenins oleanolic acid and bayogenin, contribute to its activity.

Oregon grape (*Berberis aquifolium,* also called *Mahonia aquifolium*) root is another useful urinary tract antiseptic. Its alkaloid berberine possesses wide antimicrobial activity against bacteria including Staph., Strep., and E. coli, fungus including Candida, and protozoa such as Entamoeba. In tests on Strep. and E. coli strains that cause urinary tract infections berberine reduced their ability to stick to the type of cells that line the tract. In addition to jatrorrhizine, another root alkaloid, berberine has demonstrated anti-inflammatory activity.

Narrow-leafed **echinacea** (*Echinacea angustifolia*) root is useful for infections throughout the body. It is especially appropriate in cases where there is a tendency towards chronic or repeated infections which are common in the urinary tract. Echinacea helps increase resistance by stimulating the immune response. This immune modulation is due to its isobutylamides and the phenolics echinacoside and cynarin.

Marshmallow (*Althea officinalis*) root is known for its soothing demulcent effect on the inner linings of the respiratory, digestive, and urinary tracts. The root contains sugars attached to uronic acid which forms a mucilage when extracted that coats the linings of hollow organs. This potentiates the effect of other anti-inflammatory substances.

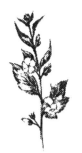

To keep the urine diluted and prevent prolonged retention it is desirable to consume more fluids than what thirst demands. This herbal combination is most effective in an alkaline medium, so it should not be used with either cranberry juice or with large amounts of vitamin C. It is also important to avoid consuming sugars that pass into the urine and feed the bacteria, whether they be from candy, desserts, sodas, or even honey and fruit juices. Marshmallow root tea can provide a soothing diuretic drink with a pleasant flavor for use as a vehicle by soaking the ground root in water overnight to extract more of the mucilage.

Add one of the following formulas if needed.

Prostate Tonic Formula

In cases in men where the prostate gland is enlarged it can block the flow of urine and prevent the complete emptying of the bladder. The retained urine can be fertile ground for bacterial growth. Until the prostate problem is resolved it is helpful to periodically use a urinary antiseptic to avoid developing an infection.

Heart Tonic Formula

Heart tonics and vasodilators help insure good blood flow to the kidneys so that the body does not retain water and waste. The reduction of fluid retention is also important to control high blood pressure and the strain it causes on the heart. As long as potassium is supplied and sodium is restricted in the diet, stimulating fluid excretion through the kidneys with diuretics is a useful temporary means of accomplishing this.

URINARY EXCRETION FACILITATION

KIDNEY AND BLADDER IRRITANTS

Concentrated Urine   Bacteruria
Extreme Urinary pH   Glycosuria
Crystal Aggregation   Trauma
Urine Retention

AGENTS THAT PROTECT THE KIDNEYS AND BLADDER

Cleansing Diuretics	Urinary Antiseptics	Antilithics	Hemostatics	Anti-inflammatories
Water Horsetail Goldenrod	Cranberry Uva Ursi Oregon Grape Echinacea	Horsetail	Horsetail Goldenrod	Uva Ursi Oregon Grape Marshmallow

IV

BREATHING

Nose, Sinuses And Lungs

Proper breathing begins by drawing air through the nose. When there is a nasal discharge, the air passages need to be kept open. Deep breathing techniques cleanse the lungs, aid in the expulsion of mucus, and give an internal massage to abdominal organs. The avoidance of airborne irritants and strengthening immune resistance helps prevent or control many common respiratory problems. Improving ventilation, inhibiting germs, promoting mucus expulsion, or relieving coughs helps improve most of these conditions.

The importance of breath is apparent, but like most bodily functions it is taken for granted. We can survive weeks without food, days without water, but only minutes without breathing. **The inhalation of air, the exchange in the lungs of oxygen from the air for carbon dioxide from the blood, and the exhalation of the carbon dioxide is what is typically understood as respiration.** A closer look at the parts involved helps us understand and appreciate their contribution to the process. The breath should be drawn in through the nose. The nose with its chambers is designed to filter out particles and bacteria with tiny hairs and the sticky mucus covering the ridges of its inner surfaces. These trapped particles are eventually expelled by a natural slow movement of the mucus outward or by sudden involuntary sneezing or intentional blowing. The inhaled air is warmed and moistened as it passes into the highly vascular sinuses. These are located in the face and at the base of the brain adjacent to the pituitary, the master gland of the endocrine system. **The occlusion of the naso-sinus airway or habitual mouth breathing prevents the filtration, warming, and moistening of the air.** This can help lead to infections of the lungs.

It is important in conditions with inflamed membranes of the upper respiratory tract to keep the air passages free of accumulated mucus that can cover the membrane lining or block sinus openings. If the sinuses become occluded a severe infection may develop. Using humidifiers or vaporizers to add moisture to the air is an important measure to prevent the mucus from drying and adhering to the membranes. Its expulsion can be improved by regular nasal douching with tepid salt water (1/4 tsp table salt per cup of water) or mild herbal tea such as eyebright. Adding bicarbonate of soda (1/4 tsp baking soda) to the tepid salt water makes an even better nonirritating, alkaline solution for dissolving mucus. These solutions can be snuffed into the nose until they begin to trickle into the throat. The fluid is then blown out through the nose and the washing is repeated a number of times until the passages are cleansed and open for easy breathing. Hot compresses over the nose and sinuses will help promote drainage between douches. In a clinical setting the sympatho-nasal technique or bilateral nasal specifics may be indicated in severe cases of congestion or occlusion. While immune support increases resistance to infections, capsules of freeze-dried stinging nettle leaves have been found to be helpful in reducing the nasal congestion associated with hay fever. Air filters in the home can remove many respiratory allergens.

As the breath is drawn passively into the lungs, the mucus covering the air tubes in the lungs traps inhaled particles and bacteria and is slowly moved out by waves of minute hairs. **When breathing remains shallow, the elimination of contaminated mucus and the exchange of metabolic gases and stagnant air in the lungs for fresh air are not as efficient as they should be.** The regular practice of taking full, complete breaths helps to improve oxygenation and to effectively clear gaseous waste by enhancing both inspiration and expiration. This is done actively by pushing down the diaphragm, the large muscle below the lungs. This fills the lower lungs and causes the ribs to rise and abdominal wall to come forward. Then the rib cage is further expanded by drawing out the breastbone and chest. Finally, protruding the upper chest and slightly raising the shoulders allows the upper lungs to fill with air. The air is then exhaled slowly and completely, drawing the abdomen in and up, relaxing the chest, and lowering the shoulders. To actively loosen mucus and expel trapped particles, lightly tap with the fingertips over the entire rib cage while holding the breath in. Then briefly pat the chest with cupped palms while releasing the breath. The exhalation is then done rapidly and forcefully through the mouth all at once or in short puffs. This helps to clear and move the contaminated mucus up through the airways and out.

The abdominal portion of deep breathing has another action which is generally unappreciated. As the diaphragm contracts to begin the breath, it gently compresses the liver, pancreas, kidneys, and spleen which lie beneath it. This drains the venous blood out of these organs. Upon exhalation the reduction in pressure replenished the organs as they are supplied with fresh arterial blood. **The regular cleansing and nourishing massage of the abdominal organs by the diaphragm during deep breathing promotes their functions of digestion, filtration, elimination, and immune function.** For the unathletic, even for the bedridden or paralytic, the practice of abdominal breathing can provide these benefits which are usually only associated with the deep breathing that occurs during vigorous exercise.

The ease of breathing is reduced when outside influences interfere with respiratory efficiency. Air pollution is ubiquitous in modern cities and industrial areas. Habitual cigarette smoking is epidemic in our society. Because of the rapid absorption of nicotine, smoking tobacco affects not only the respiratory tract but the entire system. But the greatest damage from the irritants, tars, and cancer-causing agents in the smoke is directly to the lungs. Partial protection from lung damage can be provided by the consumption of vitamin C and carotenes. **For respiratory health it is essential that habitual smoking and unnecessarily exposure to inhaled toxins be eliminated.** Allergens, such as pollens, mold spores, and danders, are other factors that can adversely affect breathing. Asthma, the narrowing of bronchial tubes that channel air into the lungs, is often a reaction to allergens or irritants such as secondary tobacco smoke that cause respiratory distress. This requires the use of antispasmodic bronchodilators (substances that open the air passages in the lungs wider) to improve the ventilation of the lungs. Avoiding the allergens and irritants and reducing the lung's sensitivity helps to prevent these attacks.

Infections are the most common acute cause of breathing difficulties. Exposure to infections is especially threatening for smokers and asthmatics whose conditions also make them more susceptible. Viral infections are particularly problematic since they cannot be eliminated by antibiotics and often lead to serious secondary bacterial infections. Controlling viral respiratory infections should be accompanied by measures to prevent these bacterial complications. Aromatic vapors in steam provide some antiseptic activity that is directed at the respiratory passages. **Besides inhibiting the growth of the germs, both viral and bacterial infections can also be approached by enhancing immune function.**

The increased production or reduced clearing of mucus from the lungs aggravates infections and asthma. Tobacco smoking especially hampers the normal removal of mucus by reducing the number of fine hairs in the bronchial tubes that help move it out. **Excessive mucus can be addressed with herbal expectorants (promote the expulsion of mucus from the lungs) and antispasmodic bronchodilators.** Together with deep breathing and inhaling aromatic vapors in steam to liquify mucus, these agents and methods help to aerate the entire lung and speed recovery from infections. Postural drainage with percussive massage over the lungs is another beneficial measure that can be used, except in cases of high blood pressure. The deep, penetrating heat from clinical diathermy treatments is helpful to improve circulation in the lungs. **Anyone suffering from pneumonia or expelling green-, red- or rust-colored sputum should be under the care of a physician.**

Coughing can be helpful when it clears excessive mucus from the lungs. This is called a productive cough. When the air passages are dry or coughing is persistent, it irritates the membrane lining these passages. This aggravates the sensitive surfaces and worsens the condition. **Obtaining relief from the cough becomes important, especially at night when it interferes with necessary sleep.** In this situation the membranes and nerves in the throat and lungs need to be soothed and relaxed.

Breathe Freely Formula

The feelings of anxiety that accompany an asthma attack literally leave one breathless. When stress is a factor in bringing on asthma attacks, the following relaxant nervine herbs may help prevent the symptoms or reduce their severity. The sedative, antispasmodic, and expectorant properties of herbs in this formula are indicated for the symptoms associated with mild to moderate asthma. Asthma is often associated with chronic exposure to tobacco smoke, especially during childhood.

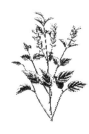

Skullcap (*Scutellaria lateriflora*) tops have a reputation for calming agitated mental conditions including those associated with withdrawal such as the DTs (delirium tremens of alcoholism). It has been used as a nervine where there is excitability or restlessness with associated insomnia. It also has been valued as a muscular antispasmodic for nervous conditions.

Fresh, immature **oat** (*Avena sativa*) seeds have also been known for their mild muscular antispasmodic and calming nervine effects. They are especially good for debility and nervous exhaustion from chronic conditions. Extracts of the green, milky seeds have been used and studied for several different addictions. Clinical trials have shown both tobacco and opium/morphine use is reduced when the extract is administered to addicts. It has also been recommended for alcohol dependance. Tests indicate that it antagonizes the effects of both nicotine and morphine.

Lobelia (*Lobelia inflata*) leaves and seeds provide potent bronchial antispasmodic and expectorant activity. Lobelia is best known for its use in asthma and respiratory conditions with excessive mucus secretions. **However, it will cause vomiting if taken in excessive dosages.** Its action is primarily due to the alkaloid lobeline that is most concentrated in its flowers and seeds. The lobeline binds to nicotinic receptors and acts by mimicking or antagonizing nicotine, depending on the organ. In a test of brain receptors it was found that lobeline is a strong competitor for the receptors that cause the mind to recognize nicotine. Several studies using lobeline as a smoking deterrent showed a decrease in the number of cigarettes smoked by those who continued. It also increased significantly the number of smokers who stopped completely.

Yerba santa (*Eriodictyon californicum*) leaves are fragrant and covered with a thick resin. Their pleasant flavor led to the official recognition of Aromatic Syrup of Eriodictyon in the *National Formulary VI* as a vehicle to mask the taste of bitter remedies. Extracts are also used as an expectorant and bronchial antispasmodic for asthma, colds, and other respiratory infections with excessive mucus production. The leaves contain an active antibacterial principle called eriodin that is effective against gram-positive and tuberculosis bacteria. The resin is rich in flavonoids of which derivatives of eriodictyol such as homoeriodictyol are the most prominent.

Licorice (*Glycyrrhiza glabra*) root is a soothing demulcent expectorant and flavorful addition to any

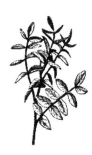

combination. In fact, not only is licorice extract used as a flavoring agent in vehicles for medicine, but many tobacco products are also flavored with licorice. Certain of the sapogenin or flavonoid components of licorice inhibit tumor promoters like those found in tobacco smoke. Some of these constituents have anti-inflammatory or antimicrobial activity. When diluted in combinations it is safe to use for a prolonged period, but it would be best to supplement potassium and methionine if it is used long-term. **High blood pressure or heart failure prohibit the continual use of large amounts of licorice because of possible fluid retention and potassium loss.**

The habitual use of tobacco is a major cause of many preventable health problems. The tobacco habit in some smokers can be broken by reducing the urge to smoke and allaying the effects of withdrawal. This process can be made somewhat easier when physiological aids are employed. These same influences can also be beneficial for other disruptive addictions such as desire for opiates. Breaking patterns of repetitive behavior is difficult even when addictive substances are not involved. Methods ranging from prayer, meditation, counselling, and hypnotherapy to acupuncture, hydrotherapy techniques, breathing exercises, and nutritional supplements can further contribute to a desirable outcome.

Add the following formula if needed.

Cough Relief and Expectorant Formula

It is important to relieve the trapping of mucus to fully restore the complete respiratory capacity. Certain herbs in the expectorant formula have antispasmodic properties that further enhance the effect desired by asthmatics. For those with a chronic smoke-induced cough the best thing next to removing the cause is to cleanse the air passages of tars and other irritants through expectoration. Broncho-dilating herbs help to keep these passages fully open.

Antiviral and Antibacterial Formula

The common cold and the flu are two illnesses which frustrate people most because of their prevalence and viral nature. These troublesome infections produce congestion and mucus discharges from both the upper and lower respiratory tract. They run rampant in the winter months. Antibiotics are ineffective in treating them. The usual over-the-counter remedies that are available for treating symptoms do not improve the course of the disease. Simple measures such as rest, the generous consumption of clear fluids, and immune support from nutritional supplements are the standards of home care. These help avoid the need for most medical intervention in overcoming the sickness. The use of the following herbs that inhibit viral growth, help prevent bacterial complications, strengthen the immune response, and reduce spasms are additionally advantageous.

Lomatium (*Lomatium dissectum,* formerly called *Leptotaenia dissecta*) root is a native American remedy that was used both as a food and for lung diseases. Its extract was introduced to more widespread use after its noteworthy benefits for the flu during the epidemic of 1917. It has been shown to contain antimicrobial tetronic acid and flavonoid components that inhibit bacteria and fungus. Its three similar coumarin glycosides include columbianin which is a potent agent for reducing smooth muscle spasms.

Osha (*Ligusticum porteri*) root is another native American herb that was used for bacterial and viral lung infections, as an expectorant for bronchial problems, and for pain. Its extract actively inhibits the growth of some bacteria and yeast. Its major constituent is ligustilide which is a phthalide having spasm-relieving activity.

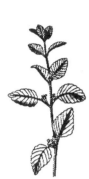

Lemon balm (*Melissa officinalis*) leaves and extracts have been used as gentle sedatives and antispasmodics. They have shown antiviral activity in a number of tests, due in part to their caffeic and rosmarinic acid content. The extract also has demonstrated immune stimulating activity. Its aromatic oil has shown broad antibacterial and antifungal effects and provides also the sedative and antispasmodic activity. When taken warm, lemon balm is useful as a diaphoretic to help increase perspiration.

Yarrow (*Achillea millefolium*) flowers have also been used as an antispasmodic and diaphoretic when the hot extract is used. It was frequently taken for colds, the flu, and fevers. Its flavonoids are mostly responsible for the antispasmodic activity and the aromatic oils contribute to its diaphoretic, febrifuge, and expectorant properties.

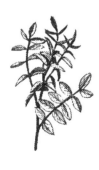

Licorice (*Glycyrrhiza glabra*) root has been used as a soothing expectorant for common bronchial problems and hoarseness. It contains the triterpenoid glycyrrhizin which inhibits viral growth and augment the immune response by inducing interferon. Its aglycone glycyrrhetic acid is both antiviral and antitussive. A number of licorice isoflavonoids have shown antimicrobial activity. The flavor and demulcent quality of licorice also improve the tolerance of bitter herbal formulas. When diluted in combinations it is safe to use, but **continual use is contraindicated in cases of high blood pressure or heart failure.**

Vegetable glycerine added to this herbal combination gives it a sweet taste and soothing sensation. The formula should be taken at the usual dose three times per day in warm water. Its use as diaphoretic remedy for increasing perspiration to help control a fever requires that it be taken in a warm beverage.

Add one of the following formulas if needed.

Immune Support Formula

In all infections, but most especially in infections caused by viruses, it is important that resistance by the immune system is optimal. Immune support helps antiseptics and antibiotics overcome bacterial invaders. For virus-caused illnesses strengthening the immune response is in many cases the best approach to treatment.

Cough Relief and Expectorant Formula

While overcoming viral respiratory infections it is desirable to obtain symptomatic relief for the more aggravating symptoms. Helping to expel mucus and reducing the intensity or frequency of a cough leads to more rapid resolution. When dealing with a cough caused by viral infection, preventing bacterial involvement should also be addressed.

Children's Calming Elixir Formula

When the fever of influenza is associated with restlessness and dry skin there is a need for herbs that can calm the distress and increase sweating. Such combinations should then be taken in warm water. The flavor of an elixir helps to make the taste of another formula acceptable to children. The aromatics also aid in the fight against respiratory infections.

Cough Relief and Expectorant Formula

The clearance of accumulated mucus and microbes from the air passages is important in respiratory tract infections. This is more difficult for the lungs than for the nose and sinuses. It is typically

done by coughing, but this can itself become debilitating. Methods and means that make it easier help
conserve energy and prevent further irritation of
tissues that are already inflamed. Aromatic oils from
plants are commonly used expectorants, agents that
promote expulsion of mucus from the air passages of
the lungs. Increasing bronchial fluid secretions with
expectorants helps to liquify the mucus and make it
more mobile. Antispasmodic bronchodilators widen
the passages through which the mucus and air must
travel. In cases where there is a dry, irritable cough
caused by tight and sensitive passages with diminished mucus, the expectorants and antispasmodics
have a soothing and relaxing antitussive effect (reducing the tendency to cough). Herbs that help control
the edema in the lungs improve the recovery. Those
that inhibit the microbes that cause the changes in
fluid and mucus output are additionally beneficial.

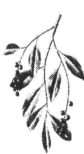

Wild cherry (*Prunus serotina*) bark is a long-time
favorite in cough remedies because of its reputed
sedative effect on respiratory nerves that initiate
coughing. Its aromatic oil is credited with this
property. The green bark also contains the cyanide-
releasing compound prunasin. The small amount of
cyanide released causes a reflex stimulation of the
respiratory center and increases the rate of breathing.
**Though wild cherry bark is safe when small quanti-
ties are taken as part of an herbal combination, it
must not be used in large amounts.**

Licorice (*Glycyrrhiza glabra*) root is commonly
used for respiratory conditions with coughing,
hoarseness, and mucus congestion. It is both demulcent and expectorant. Its isoflavonoids are antimicrobial. The component glycyrrhizin has both antiviral
and immune-enhancing effects. Also, its aglycone
glycyrrhetic acid has central cough suppressant

effects that are as potent as codeine. The flavor is an
additional benefit in combinations. It is safe for
periodic use in acute cases, especially when diluted,
but **licorice should not be continually used in cases of
high blood pressure or heart failure.**

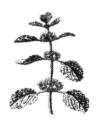

Horehound (*Marrubium vulgare*) leaves are
principally used as an antitussive for coughs and as an
expectorant to improve secretions in bronchitis. This
effect is due to the monoterpenes in its aromatic oil.
Horehound extracts also inhibit smooth muscle
contractions caused by serotonin.

Red clover (*Trifolium pratense*) blossoms have
traditionally been used to relieve spasmodic coughs
and as an expectorant. Red clover polysaccharides
can lead to local white blood cell accumulation.

Elecampane (*Inula helenium*) root is another
expectorant remedy whose aromatic oil is beneficial
in bronchitis with mucus congestion and coughing.
Helenin, a mixture of mostly alantolactones, makes
up a major portion of this oil. Helenin inhibits the
growth of many nonviral microorganisms.

White pine (*Pinus strobus*) bark is another
familiar ingredient used in remedies for coughs and
colds. Its oleoresin supplies another source of expectorant aromatic oils.

Poplar (*Populus balsamifera*) buds are used for
cough relief as an expectorant for respiratory congestion. They contain a balsamic resin whose major
terpenoid component is likely the anti-inflammatory
bisabolol. The salicin content gives mild aspirin-like
relief for fever and inflammation. Dihydrochalcone
flavonoids, the major constituents of the bud exudate,
inhibit inflammatory secretions from immune system cells.

Fennel (*Foeniculum vulgare*) seeds are used to
relieve coughing. Their aromatic constituent anethole has expectorant effects. They also contain cholin-

ergic activators that can help improve the fluid quality of the mucus.

Gumweed (*Grindelia robusta*) flowers have a history of use for the inflammation and constriction of the bronchial tubes. This is due to their expectorant and bronchial antispasmodic properties. The expectorant activity has been demonstrated in cats but not in other lab animals. The flowers produce a resinous exudate with a balsamic odor that is extracted in alcohol. The resin contains grindelic acid and related diterpene acid derivatives.

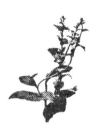

Lobelia (*Lobelia inflata*) leaves and seeds are important sources of an antispasmodic bronchodilator compound. These provide the alkaloid lobeline along with similar alkaloids. The lobeline acts as a respiratory stimulant and has been shown to protect against edema in the lungs. **Lobelia can cause vomiting in large doses.**

Lomatium (*Lomatium dissectum*, formerly called *Leptotaenia dissecta*) root was used in lung disease for its antimicrobial properties produced in part by its tetronic acid and flavonoid constituents. One of its coumarin glycosides, columbianin, has been shown to have potent antispasmodic activity.

Bitter orange (*Citrus vulgaris,* also called *C. aurantium*) peel aromatic oil has been used for chronic bronchial inflammation. It also has some antibacterial activity. Its flavor and antiseptic action are due in part to its high limonene content.

A vegetable glycerin base provides a sweet, syrup-like, soothing effect without using sugar. The combination of aromatic compounds produces a pleasant flavor that is agreeable to children. It should be taken in the usual dose three times per day, especially at bedtime.

Add one of the following formulas if needed.

Immune Support Formula

When coughs are the result of an infectious process, treating the cause involves strengthening resistance to the infection. This should be done in addition to any medical approach that specifically inhibits the growth of the particular germ involved in the infection.

Breathe Freely Formula

In "wet coughs" in which a lot of mucus is expelled, additional expectorants are helpful to assist in its expulsion. Antispasmodic expectorants that act to dilate the bronchial tubes are especially beneficial to help clear the mucus from the lungs. Even in dry coughs the antispasmodic herbs help to relax the bronchial tightness and can relieve an irritable cough somewhat.

Antiviral and Antibacterial Formula

Coughs that are caused by bronchial infections such as colds, the flu, or bronchitis can benefit from herbs that help to control the growth of germs. Respiratory infections that involve the lung itself and threaten breathing require examination by a physician and possibly antibiotics if caused by bacteria. (Such cases of bacterial pneumonia requiring a doctor typically include fever and discolored sputum that is expelled by coughing.)

PROMOTING EFFICIENT BREATHING

HEALTH OF THE LUNGS

Disease Susceptibility Factors	Protective Approaches	Aiding Contaminant Expulsion
Mouth Breathing	Nasal Breathing	Forceful Exhalations
Shallow Breathing	Nasal Douching	Expectorants
Nasal /Sinus Catarrh	Deep Breathing	Bronchodilators
Tobacco Smoke	Filtering the Air	Light Tapping Over
Air -Pollution	Full Breathing	Lungs
Exposure to Infections	Avoiding Smoke-	Aromatic Vaporization
Allergens	filled Rooms	Postural Drainage
	Vitamin C	Diathermy
	Carotenes	Coughing
	Aromatic	Eliminate Smoking
	Vaporization	Habit
	Enhancing	
	Immunity	

RESPIRATORY RELIEF AGENTS

Asthma	Bronchitis	Coughs

Bronchodilators:
Lobelia
Yerba Santa

Nervines:
Skullcap
Green Oats

Expectorants:
Lobelia
Yerba Santa
Licorice

Antimicrobials:
Lomatium
Osha
Lemon Balm
Licorice

Expectorants:
Yarrow
Licorice
Osha

Antitussives:
Wild Cherry
Licorice
Horehound
Red Clover

Antimicrobials:
Lomatium
Elecampane
Licorice
Bitter Orange

Expectorants:
Gumweed
Lobelia
Licorice
Horehound
Red Clover
Elecampane
White Pine
Poplar
Fennel

Bronchodilators:
Gumweed
Lobelia

V

CIRCULATION

Heart And Blood Vessels

The delivery of blood to living tissues is neces-
sary for their normal function. The primary means of
insuring adequate circulation is by maintaining
proper exercise, relaxation, and diet. Several legal
drugs from plants can be involved in causing certain
cardiac and circulatory problems.

The heart is a muscle and regular aerobic activity
is needed in order to optimize its ability to pump
blood. The arterial blood vessels are dynamic chan-
nels through which the blood is delivered in order to
carry nutrients to all the tissues in the body. If the
blood flow is forced through narrow vascular chan-
nels, the heart has to strain harder to pump against
the resistance. Regular relaxation helps the vessels to
better dilate (open wide). Alternating exercise and
relaxation enables the heart to bring the vital nourishment contained in the blood to its own tissue and
to the rest of the body. **To accomplish this requires**
blood vessels that can accommodate changing local
needs. The chronic presence of excessive fats and
sugar in the blood is detrimental to the elasticity of
the vessels. The adequate consumption of other
nutrients including certain minerals and flavonoids is

important for maintaining the functional integrity of the blood vessels. So balanced nutrition is paramount to assure the health not only of tissues throughout the body but of the circulatory system itself.

To improve heart strength it is not necessary to do the exercises required to develop large muscle mass or to undergo endurance training. The ordinary exertion required for brisk walking, cycling, cross-country skiing, or swimming is adequate to increase the heart's tone and capacity if done regularly. **By raising the heart rate through moderate exercise the circulation of the heart itself is improved, and its reserve capacity to deliver more blood to the body on demand is increased.** This takes about 30 minutes at a time for four or five days each week. Such activity is a wonderful way to begin the day. Moving about in nature stimulates the body through its active use and awakens the mind for the day ahead. Others find it beneficial to end the day with this type of routine. This can help to release pent-up thoughts and emotions and thus to prepare a tired mind and body for a restful night's sleep. It is a great advantage to be able to do both.

The importance of this type of nonstrenuous exercise is not limited to the delivery of blood. Most of the fluid that re-enters venous blood vessels or remains as lymph around the tissue cells must return to the heart against the force of gravity. This requires external pressure on these vessels by the surrounding muscles. The squeezing helps the blood and lymph to advance upward as these fluids are prevented from flowing back by one-way valves in the vessels. This process is known as the venous pump. **Exercise improves the circulation by increasing both the heart's output and the venous blood's return.**

As necessary as exercise is for the heart, conscious

relaxation is of equal importance for some. **When continual physical, mental, and/or emotional demands create chronic excessive stress, the adrenals and adrenergic nerves respond by imposing a detrimental influence on the circulation.** Adrenalin increases the heart rate while surface and visceral blood vessels narrow. This increases resistance to blood flow. The heart pumps harder to supply blood and so the blood pressure is raised. Through relaxation techniques it is possible to beneficially influence the heart rate and blood vessel tone.

One effective means to relax is by the regular practice of slow, deep breathing. This produces a cholinergic response and balances the autonomic nerve activity. **Together with slow breathing, progressive relaxation of the body dissipates the adrenergic nerve control.** While lying on the back the muscles are successively relaxed by beginning with the feet, legs, and thighs, continuing with the abdomen, chest and back, then going to the hands, forearms, arms, and shoulders, and finally to the neck, face, and around the eyes. It is best to focus on releasing those areas where most of the tension is held. This can be done while imagining a pleasant, warm, peaceful setting to provide a sense of calm. Such relaxation exercises help to slow the heart rate and lower blood pressure. Biofeedback training is another means for people to learn to consciously relax.

Nutrition is important in circulatory health both in regards to what should be eaten and what is best avoided. The emphasis on avoiding cholesterol has led to an undeserved neglect of other factors associated with developing atherosclerosis. This type of hardening of the arteries occurs with the local deposition of cholesterol and fats in the vessels. The liver produces most of the harmful cholesterol in our bodies. It does so largely in response to the consumption of excessive fat in the diet. Saturated fats from animal products and hardened vegetable oils such as margarine are particularly undesirable in cases of high cholesterol, as is sugar. In place of using saturated fats in the diet it is better to consume small amounts of vegetable oils that contain the essential unsaturated linoleic and linolenic fatty acids (for example, soy and flax seed oils, respectively). The metabolic derivatives of these essential fatty acids, GLA (found in black currant and evening primrose oils) and EPA (found in fish oils), respectively, are transformed into protective prostaglandins. These prostaglandins reduce dangerous blood lipids and the tendency of blood platelets to clump and form clots that block arteries. The deposits of fat in blood vessels of the heart and to the brain provide locations where clots can form. The amino acid carnitine helps to mobilize blood fats.

Obesity and high levels of sugar in the blood of diabetics have long been recognized as factors in developing arteriosclerosis. The various forms of this condition including atherosclerosis result in a hardening and thickening of arterial blood vessels. This leads to a reduction in local blood flow. Management of both obesity and high blood sugar through diet emphasizes the avoidance of sweets and fats and consumption of complex carbohydrates, fiber, and sources of the mineral chromium. The need for adequate calcium and magnesium to reduce vascular narrowing and improve the contractions of the heart has been established. High blood pressure is another risk factor for developing arteriosclerosis. Excessive intake of sodium from salt can increase the fluid volume and aggravate high blood pressure. Unfortunately, the diuretics that are given to reduce fluid volume and blood pressure can lower potassium and produce arrhythmias. Along with sodium restriction, generous consumption of dark green leafy vegetables provides the balance of the mineral nutrients (calcium, magnesium, and potassium) helpful in combatting high blood pressure. Additional supplementation may be necessary in pathological cases. Flavonoids and vitamin C supplied by fruits and vegetables are essential for maintaining vascular tone and integrity.

Habitual consumption of plants containing common legal stimulants should be avoided. These can interfere with the normal nerve and muscle function of the heart and blood vessels. Coffee, tea, cola and other caffeine sources and ephedra tea or hay fever, asthma, and cold remedies containing ephedrine can aggravate heart rhythm and blood pressure problems. Using tobacco products containing nicotine is likewise associated with these problems as well as other conditions involving peripheral vascular constriction.

Heart Tonic Formula

Reduced blood flow in the heart muscle follows the narrowing of its arteries from atherosclerosis. If these arteries constrict further they temporarily fail to supply the heart with enough oxygen which produces angina pectoris (pain in the chest). With generalized arteriosclerosis or excessive adrenergic tone the blood pressure is elevated, since the heart must force blood through constricted arteries. As it attempts to beat harder and faster, the heart becomes overworked. In some cases the heart does not contract with enough force. Fatigue and heavy breathing occurs after slight exertion. It compensates for this

by beating faster. Digitalis and its glycosides are
frequently used to increase the strength of heart
contractions and to reduce the heart rate. However,
they are quite toxic, and in cases with angina pectoris
or arrhythmias they can be dangerous to use.
Arrhythmias can arise from the influence of caffeine
and nicotine, but at times they may also be caused by
diminished circulation in the heart. This combination uses herbs that help relax the vessels through
which the blood is pumped, and includes a plant with
moderate tonic effects to support the heart contractions. These effects help to relieve the strain on the
heart and control blood pressure. The increased
blood supply to the heart helps prevent angina and
arrhythmias. **However, it remains necessary for any
one with symptoms of heart disease to be under the
care of a physician for their condition.**

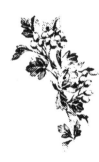

Hawthorn (*Crataegus oxyacantha* and/or *C.
monogyna*) berries, flowers, and leaves have been
used for degenerative conditions of the heart associated with coronary arteriosclerosis because of their
unique vasodilating effect. Blood flow to the heart
tissue is increased, angina pectoris can be relieved,
and arrhythmias are prevented with the persistent use
of hawthorn or its extracts. Blood pressure can be
improved also, since peripheral blood flow is somewhat increased. Though hawthorn has only a mild
tonic effect on the heart, when used with cardiac
glycoside drugs their effect is improved and their
toxicity is reduced. Cardiac tonic amines including
tyramine are contained in the flowers, as well as
hyperoside and other flavonoids. The hawthorn
leaves have flavan polymers of epicatechol, while the
fruit and leaves contain the flavonoid vitexin and its
glycosides. Oligomeric procyanidins are present
throughout. Its flavan polymers increase heart tone

and lower blood pressure, as does the flavonoid mixture. Hawthorn's flavonoids also improve blood flow. The flavonoid mixture improves collateral circulation of the heart after vascular blockage and aids in recovery. Vitexin protects against vascular spasms, high blood pressure, rapid heart rate, and arrhythmias. The procyanidin polymers from hawthorn improve blood flow to the heart and lower blood pressure. The combined effects of all the components are even greater than their added individual activities.

Fresh **cactus** (*Cactus grandiflorus,* also called *Selenicereus grandiflorus*) flowers and stems have been used as a tonic for many functional heart conditions. These include arrhythmias, angina pectoris, enlargement, edema, and problems associated with tobacco use. **Cactus is generally contraindicated for patients with high blood pressure when used alone.** Animal research indicated that the effect of Cactus tincture on the blood pressure is not significant. The alcoholic extract was shown to increase the strength of heart contractions and reduce arrhythmias in its upper chambers. Cactus produces mild diuretic effects. In high doses it increased the heart rate. Cactus contains a number of alkaloids including hordenine. Its tyramine component was shown to increase the contractile force of the heart.

Passion flower (*Passiflora incarnata*) leaves are commonly thought of as a sedative antispasmodic. They have been used for both cardiac pain and palpitations. Like hawthorn the leaves contain the flavonoid vitexin, but fresh leaves also have large amounts of its isomer isovitexin and the flavonoid orientin. While vitexin lowers blood pressure and is antispasmodic, orientin and vitexin both protect against arrhythmias and reduced blood flow to the heart.

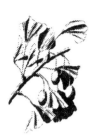

Extracts of **ginkgo** (*Ginkgo biloba*) leaves are effective peripheral vasodilators for circulatory problems in the extremities. They also protect against insufficient blood flow in the brain. In addition, the extracts increase blood flow to the heart muscle, thereby protecting against cardiac arrhythmias. This vasodilating activity is due in part to flavonol glycosides of quercetin, kaempferol, and isorhamnetin that are unique to ginkgo. Pro-anthocyanidins are also active constituents. Still other active components are the unique terpenes called ginkgolides. These inhibit clumping of plate-lets caused by platelet activating factor that can clog narrowed arteries. Ginkgo extract also antagonizes the reduction of blood flow to the heart muscle that is caused by platelet activating factor.

This combination should be taken three times each day in the usual dosage for adults (15 - 30 drops). The herbs in this combination that dilate blood vessels affect blood pressure by reducing resistance from constricted vessels. This modifies the potential effect of Cactus of raising the blood pres-sure which might occur if Cactus were used by itself. The diuretic effect of Cactus may help reduce high blood pressure in cases caused by increased blood volume from fluid retention.

Add one of the following formulas if needed.

Diuretic and Urinary Antiseptic Formula

If high blood pressure is associated with fluid retention, the use of diuretics can help by reducing the volume of blood. Steps must then be taken to replace potassium lost due to the diuresis. If fluid retention is determined by clinical examination to be the result of congestive heart failure, the physician must determine the most appropriate medication for strengthening heart contractions.

Mental Energy Formula

For those who are aged and suffer from reduced mental function in conjunction with poor heart strength, the need for improving the brain's metabolism and circulation cannot be overemphasized. A variety of symptoms due to inefficient nerve activity may respond to increasing the flow of blood and nourishment to the brain.

Balanced Blood Formula

Those with circulatory problems, the overweight, and others who need to control fat and/or sugar levels must protect their arteries from damage. Measures to prevent arteriosclerosis are essential so that many heart and vascular problems can be avoided.

Balanced Blood Formula

Because of dietary indiscretion or metabolic dysfunction the levels of blood sugar or cholesterol are elevated beyond the proper range for many in our society. The potential medical problems faced by diabetics if their sugar level is not controlled are disturbing. These problems include arteriosclerosis, kidney failure, nerve damage, and blindness. It is vital to control blood sugar levels before any of these conditions develop. High blood cholesterol is also associated with an increased risk of arteriosclerosis and coronary heart disease. The secondary effects of high blood sugar and cholesterol are too numerous to discuss. It is necessary that the diet be properly managed to prevent elevated levels of these compounds in the blood. This formula can be another aid to control mild elevations in blood sugar and/or cholesterol levels. This is especially advantageous early in the course of their development. If these steps are inadequate for some individuals then other medicine or supplements must be employed to reduce the elevated levels. Even then the continuance of supportive measures is desirable. **Only under medical supervision and monitoring should any attempt be made by diabetics on insulin to reduce blood sugar levels.**

Fenugreek (*Trigonella foenum-graecum*) seeds have been used largely as a demulcent. They have recently been found to reduce the undesirable forms of cholesterol and fats in the blood of patients who have high levels. Using fenugreek did not alter the beneficial forms of cholesterol in the blood. The reduction is due to both its fiber and saponin content. The saponins diosgenin and tigogenin helped lower the blood cholesterol in diabetic and non-diabetic animals. There is also a lowering of blood sugar levels by the fiber content in diabetic animals. This aids in preventing the development of high blood cholesterol. Its coumarin component lowers blood sugar in animals that are diabetic and non-diabetic. The fenugreek alkaloid trigonelline can also lower blood sugar significantly as shown in rats and some diabetic patients.

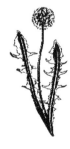

Dandelion (*Taraxacum officinale*) leaves and roots are used for their cholagogue and diuretic effects. By increasing fluid loss and reducing blood volume diuretics help take strain off of the heart. However, unlike other diuretics which lead to potassium loss that can cause arrhythmias, dandelion supplies potassium which helps protect the heart. While the leaves are more potent as a diuretic, the root is better for stimulating the liver secretory activity. Besides reducing liver congestion, extracts lower cholesterol levels in the blood, probably by its producing an increased output of bile. Dandelion can also lower blood sugar content.

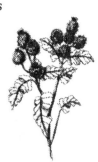

Burdock (*Arctium lappa*) seeds are mostly used as a diuretic. They contain the compounds arctiin and arctigenin which are used for treating kidney disorders. Its lignans components including trachelogenin lower high blood pressure by their calcium antagonistic activity. The root of burdock is also used. Its extract has demonstrated a long-lasting reduction in blood sugar content and increased carbohydrate tolerance.

Devil's club (*Oplopanax horridum*, formerly called *Fatsia horrida*) root bark extract with its tannins removed has been shown to lower blood sugar. The hypoglycemic principle is insoluble in a neutral or alkaline solution. It is nontoxic when given orally and works best when fresh vegetables are included in the diet. Water extracts of the root bark also contain an element which raises blood sugar. Consequently, several studies could show no overall lowering of the blood sugar when using alkaline or crude extracts. The hypoglycemic principle can be separated by precipitation using acetone. Due to inconsistent results this herb taken by itself should not be relied upon.

Huckleberry (*Vaccinium myrtilis*, also called bilberry or blueberry) leaves and berries are considered astringent and antiseptic. The leaves contain the antiseptic compounds ursolic acid and hydroquinone, more tannins, and hydroxyflavans such as epicatechin, while the fruit yields more anthocyanosides of delphinidin and cyanidin. Neomyrtillin (7 methyl-delphinidin) is the active component from a huckleberry leaf extract (myrtillin) that lowers blood sugar. Myrtillin is extracted in alcohol to separate it from another component that raises blood sugar. Myrtillin also reduces sugar in the urine and aids wound healing in diabetics. A water and alcohol extract of the leaves can also lower blood fat (triglyceride) and cholesterol levels. The anthocyanosides of delphinidin and cyanidin have an affinity for skin and kidney tissue. These anthocyanosides have a protective effect on small blood vessels by strengthening the collagen in vessel walls. This reduces excessive leakage from the vessels into tissues due to high blood pressure. These anthocyanosides reduce platelet clumping and relax contractions in blood vessels by stimulating production of specific prostaglandins. In diabetics they help prevent aneurysms from developing in the small vessels of the eyes.

The use of oral nutritional and herbal supplements to lower blood sugar and cholesterol is a convenient approach. However, in cases of diabetes they cannot be expected to completely replace the dependency on medicine such as insulin injections. In no case should insulin use be abruptly discontinued to try another agent on a trial basis. Coma or death can result from such an imprudent choice. As an alternative method for lowering cholesterol such substitution is not as acutely risky. The use of any such remedy as a means to indulge one's appetite and attempt to avoid the consequences is completely inappropriate. There must be compliance to a program of proper nutrition to avoid aggravating a condition that already exists. Such dietary management can often prevent problems from developing to begin with.

Add one of the following formulas if needed.

Heart Tonic Formula

If circulation is compromised due to deposits or fibrotic constriction of the blood vessels in the extremities, herbs that help to dilate the arteries and increase blood flow will aid greatly in reducing potential problems. The improved blood flow is essential for peripheral tissues to improve their functioning by bringing necessary nutrients and to remain healthy by facilitating removal of metabolic wastes. Simply put, stagnation of the blood is avoided.

Mental Energy Formula

Elderly individuals whose dietary habits have resulted in deposits of fats in blood vessels that serve the brain need to halt this development. The formation of clots and breakdown of normal fluid exchange in the brain can be averted by reducing risk factors and strengthening vessel walls. Improving the circulation and metabolism in brain tissue helps to overcome problems in mental function complicated by chronic degeneration.

Venous Tonic Formula

Veins, the blood vessels that carry blood back to the heart, have fewer smooth muscle fibers in their walls to maintain tone than do arteries. The back-pressure caused by a weak heart, prolonged standing, straining, pregnancy, or congestive conditions of the liver reduces the return of blood to the heart. This causes the veins to bulge and, as fluid leaks from the veins, produces edema. Enlarged veins are not only unsightly but can be unhealthy and uncomfortable. When back-pressure occurs in the rectal veins hemorrhoids can develop. Varicose veins occur in the legs when they become so widened that their valves cannot prevent the backflow of blood. The blood pools in the veins as they further stretch and enlarge. Aching and muscular fatigue associated with poor circulation then develops. These local symptoms result from the lack of oxygen and nutrients. As a consequence tissue repair takes longer after injuries, and skin ulcers sometimes develop. The following herbs either help to strengthen the walls of veins, increase their tone, or help prevent varicose conditions from developing or getting worse.

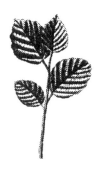

Witch hazel (*Hamamelis virginiana*) bark is astringent. It contains a tannin called hamamelitannin that dissolves in alcohol. The tannin-free extract is also slightly astringent. The extract and bark have been used internally and locally as a tonic for varicose veins and hemorrhoids. The extract is applied locally to wounds and sores to stop bleeding. Witch hazel volatile oil contains the antiseptic constituents eugenol and carvacrol.

Stoneroot (*Collinsonia canadensis*) root is best known for its use for hemorrhoids. It is also a digestive tonic, and its action includes toning the bowels and relieving constipation. This reduces the congestion and straining associated with hemorrhoids. It aids in healing other rectal sores associated with congestion and relieves the associated discomfort. Stoneroot contains the polyphenol rosmarinic acid.

Huckleberry (*Vaccinium myrtilis*) leaves contain antiseptic (hydroquinone and ursolic acid) and astringent components (tannins) while the fruit has more vasotonic constituents (hydroxyflavans and anthocyanosides). The anthocyanosides increase blood vessel resistance to leaking fluid from high blood pressure by their strengthening effect on the fibers in the vessel walls. The anthocyanosides also prevent platelet clumping that can lead to clot formation.

Rosemary (*Rosmarinus officinalis*) leaves have been used to raise the tone of blood vessels and improve overall circulation. In addition to their aromatic oil the leaves contain ursolic acid, rosmarinic acid, and a number of flavonoids. The leaves also have a derivative of rosmaricine (formed from carnosic acid) that stimulates smooth muscles and reduces pain.

Prickly ash (*Xanthoxylum,* or *Zanthoxylum, clava-herculis*) bark is used as a tonic and stimulant for sluggish circulation in cases of blood stasis with capillary engorgement. Its active components include the isobutylamide neoherculin, the lignin asarinin, and the alkaloids chelerythrine and nitidine. Chelerythrine has been shown to lower blood pressure, inhibit the breakdown of the chemical transmitter for cholinergic nerves, and inhibit inflammatory edema.

Along with the internal use of these herbs, hemorrhoids can be benefitted by external application of this extract. Internal hemorrhoids that protrude out of the anus are associated with pressure in the portal venous drainage to the liver. In this case congestion of the liver is involved and needs to be treated. External hemorrhoids under the skin of the anus involve clots that form in the bulging veins. These can result from increased venous blood pressure that occurs while straining. Warm sitz baths followed by local application of the tonic on a cotton compress helps painful external hemorrhoids. In contrast, local use of this tonic compress after cold sitz baths improves the laxity and bleeding symptoms of internal hemorrhoids.

Add the following formula if needed.

Liver Tonic Formula

In conditions of excessive venous fullness below the liver, especially in cases of hemorrhoids, back-pressure and reduced circulation due to liver congestion can aggravate the condition. By helping to improve secretions and metabolism of the liver, the congestion and bulging in lower venous blood vessels can also be relieved.

BENEFITS TO THE CARDIOVASCULAR SYSTEM

Methods and Agents	Heart	Arteries	Veins
Aerobic Exercise	•		•
Rest and Relaxation	•	•	
Deep Breathing	•	•	
Biofeedback	•	•	
Contrast Hydrotherapy		•	•
Essential Fatty Acids		•	
Carnitine	•	•	
Calcium	•	•	
Magnesium	•	•	
Green Leafy Vegetables	•	•	
Herbs			
Hawthorn	•	•	
Cactus	•		
Passion Flower	•	•	
Ginkgo	•	•	
Huckleberry		•	•
Fenugreek		•	
Devil's Club		•	
Dandelion	•	•	•
Burdock	•	•	
Stoneroot			•
Witch Hazel			•
Rosemary		•	•
Prickly Ash		•	•
Avoid			
Excess Stress	•	•	
Cholesterol	•	•	
Saturated Fats	•	•	
High Blood Sugar		•	
Obesity		•	
Excess Salt	•		
Potassium Loss	•		
Caffeine	•		
Ephedrine	•	•	
Nicotine	•	•	
Excess Standing			•
Straining			•
Liver Congestion			•

VI

MIND & MOOD

Brain And Autonomic Nerves

The power of the mind to control the body can be brought into play by the choices we make. Nerve control of body functions can be beneficially influenced by our thoughts, attitudes, and behaviors. Promoting nervous, hormonal, metabolic, and circulatory balance eases the process of adjusting to stress.

Our central nervous system (the brain and spinal cord) receives stimuli and consciously or unconsciously reacts to them. Through the brain and nerve paths we can perceive what is occurring in the world around us and interact with changing events. The marvelous network of nerves in the brain also allows us to engage in nonphysical activities that are creative and spontaneous. These mental/emotional acts can seem to be separate from physical realities, but they produce, and are strongly influenced by, chemical changes in our brains. These chemical alterations have to do not only with transmission of impulses between nerve cells and tissue but also with the availability of nutrients through the circulation.

The ability of nerves to function properly is based upon their energy metabolism and their nutrient supply. To meet the demands of ordinary stresses

requires proper circulation to provide oxygen, simple
sugar, vitamin B complex, and the minerals calcium
and magnesium. Certain amino acids from protein
are necessary precursors for impulse transmitter
substances. Depression can be associated with
reduced levels of dopamine, derived from the amino
acid tyrosine, while anxiety and wakefulness can
sometimes be improved by supplying tryptophan to
encourage serotonin production. **Without adequate
cellular nutrition the brain's perceptions can be
altered and its responses can be erratic.** Inadequate
circulation to the brain robs its cells of sufficient
nutrients. Excessive blood flow also affects the
brain's function. Daily consumption of the herb
feverfew can often prevent migraine headaches
associated with cerebral circulatory changes.

**Our body is normally controlled by electrical
messages received from the central nervous system or
the autonomic (adrenergic or cholinergic) nerves and
by chemical messages from the hormonal glands of
the body.** Thoughts of intention arising from the
cerebral cortex of the brain act through the spinal
cord to produce an immediate somatic (bodily) effect.
For example, our posture changes as we decide to
move or make our muscles become tense or relaxed.
Emotions and imagination, whether memories or
fantasies, produce unconscious somatic effects. They
are also associated with the brain's limbic system
which influences the autonomic nervous system to
alter unconscious organ functions. For example,
smelling stimulates the olfactory bulb in the limbic
system which activates feelings and memories and
changes the facial expression and heart rate. Imagination and emotions also affect the hypothalamic area
of the brain which controls many somatic and autonomic functions. In addition the hypothalamus has a

delayed control over the body's metabolic activity through chemical messages it sends to the adjacent pituitary gland. This master gland then releases hormones into the blood which act on other glands and organs throughout the body. These control levels of fluid, energy, growth, and reproductive activity over the long term by their own hormonal releases.

The attitude of a person acts as the frame of reference from which personal thoughts and emotions unfold. While emotions do not arise from conscious choice, they are influenced by the prevailing attitude. The important point to recognize is that one can cultivate positive attitudes through choice, support, and reinforcement. Doubt and insecurity are suffocating emotions. An attitude of faith benefits healing through acceptance of the therapy as a means to overcome the sickness or disease. This is conventionally called the placebo effect. It is a process in which believing that something is helpful will in itself improve the outcome. This attitude is affirmed by carefully following the chosen approach. Fear, worry, anxiety and despair are paralyzing emotions. An attitude of hope is very important, especially in cases that are prolonged or potentially terminal. Hope is the assurance that the outcome will be favorable or acceptable. It is supported by recognizing indications that progress is occurring.

Other negative emotions act differently. Anger, hate, envy, jealousy, and spite can literally gnaw at the gut. These emotions often lead to a burning desire for vengeance. This bitter attitude destroys the joy in the life of the one seeking reprisal. Not only can this attitude prolong disease, it may even cause it. The most crucial choice is to forgive by developing an attitude of love. This type of love is not the romantic emotion. Rather, it is an act of the will. Love is the decision to desire the good of another. This intention produces freedom from the need for retribution and its destructive effects. Benevolence is reinforced when it is put into practice and demonstrated. Then the emotional scars of relationships heal along with the associated physical disturbances. **These powerful attitudes of faith, hope, and love help to overcome mental, emotional, and physical problems.** One who believes in God as the ultimate source and goal of these dispositions should especially take advantage of cultivating these healing powers through prayer.

Emotions can be influenced by consciously choosing to express a certain attitude. Likewise, the unconscious control of organ functions by autonomic nerves can also be influenced through conscious choices of thoughts and/or behaviors. **The keys to influencing adrenergic and cholinergic activities are through the use of breathing, muscle tone, the surroundings, the imagination, and warm or cold water.** If there is a lack of energy or trouble focusing attention, temporarily tensing the muscles or rapidly breathing through the nose for up to one minute activates the adrenergic response. This stimulates the release of adrenalin, oxygenates the blood, excites the mind, and increases the heart rate. This technique can be replaced or enhanced by brisk walking, listening to up-tempo music or visualizing an experience of white-water rafting, skiing, or involvement in some other exciting event. For someone who is nervous and needs to calm down, slow deep breathing in a dark, quiet place can be combined with relaxing muscular tension, imagining a peaceful experience at home or in nature, or taking a stroll. This activates the cholinergic nerves which slows the heart, lowers blood pressure, and improves digestion. Hydrotherapy can enhance either effect. Warm or neutral baths act as sedative measures. Cold water sprayed over the spine, walked in, or splashed in the face is mentally and physically stimulating. By using techniques such as these the need for chemical intervention can be avoided.

Modern living can produce a great deal of stress due to the demands that confront people each day. After continually rising to meet the requirements of a fast-paced lifestyle people may reach the stage where they no longer feel capable of responding adequately to their daily responsibilities. This stage of adrenal exhaustion follows chronic adrenergic over-stimulation. **Besides the various lifestyle adjustments and behavioral techniques that can be employed, the use of certain herbal remedies can improve the efficiency with which both the mind and the body manage stressful circumstances. This influence is many faceted and involves balancing nervous, hormonal, metabolic, and circulatory activity.** Consequently, the enhanced performance instills a sense of confidence for being able to manage problems and difficulties. At times when refreshing rest is difficult to achieve, other herbs that promote relaxation can help fulfill this need.

Mental Energy Formula

Many people who rely on stimulants like caffeinated beverages could often address their need for more energy by merely improving cerebral circulation. By periodically assuming a position with the head lower than the body (by inversion or use of a slant board) or through vigorous exercising, the increased blood flow to brain tissue provides a mental stimulus. If circulation to the brain is insufficient then all mental performance suffers. As the brain's lack of nutrition becomes chronic with age mental symptoms can be severe and associated problems develop. Seeming indifference to personal appearance and social involvement may become evident. In cases where poor cerebral circulation or energy metabolism is a factor it is impossible to maintain the optimal central nervous system function. The influence of these herbal remedies can have a significant impact on these problems. Besides affecting mental function some of these herbs support adrenal response and improve the tolerance and adaptation to stress.

Ginkgo (*Ginkgo biloba*) leaves are remarkable for the ability of their ginkgolide and flavone glycoside-containing extracts to increase local blood flow to brain tissue, particularly in cerebral arteriosclerosis. This increased circulation is also produced after arterial blockage and protects the tissues from low oxygen levels. In elderly patients with chronically insufficient circulation to the brain ginkgo extract can reduce many associated symptoms. These include dizziness, headaches, ringing in the ears, memory loss, reduced vigilance, and mood disturbances. Improvements become more significant after three months of use. In addition, ginkgo extract affects brain energy metabolism by reducing its glucose utilization when oxygen is low. As a result it reduces edema of the brain with its accompanying symptoms. Ginkgo leaf extract also affects levels of amine transmitter substances in the brain. It has been shown to be useful for some diabetic arterial diseases.

Siberian ginseng (*Eleutherococcus senticosus,* also called *Acanthopanax senticosus*) root is, as the name implies, related to ginseng and similar in its adaptogenic properties. The extract stimulates brain activity and causes a more economical release of body

energy which results in increased work output.
Siberian ginseng improves the uptake of sugar by
tissue cells. It helps in the conversion of fats to
starches in the heart when its blood supply is diminished. Siberian ginseng also improves growth rates
and immune responses under stressful conditions. It
contains a mixture of eleutherosides A-E. These
include syringin (B) and syringaresinol diglucoside
(E) which were shown to diminish stress-caused
reductions of strength, memory retrieval, and sexual
behavior. The anti-stress effect seems to derive from
its antioxidant and steroid metabolism activity on the
hypothalamus-pituitary-adrenal endocrine function.
The eleutherosides bind to corticosterone receptors,
as well as male and female steroid receptors. The
eleutherosides and other components improve
adaptation to a loss of blood flow to the brain, while
the total extract increases survival. Siberian ginseng
also produces an increase of amine nerve transmitter
substances in the brain and adrenal glands.

   Gotu kola (*Centella asiatica,* also called
Hydrocotyle asiatica) leaves do not contain caffeine
and should not be confused with the caffeine-con-
taining kola nut. Their triterpenoid glycosides
asiaticoside, madecassoside, and brahmoside reduce
adrenal corticosterone blood levels during stress.
They have been found to be useful for cognitive and
nervous disorders and vascular problems of the brain.
The glycosides have antispasmodic activity in the gut.
The leaves have traditionally been used for healing
sores and skin problems. The glycosides and their
aglycone acids stimulate the production of connective
tissue ground substance. The extract also strengthens
weakened veins by enhancing collagen synthesis in
their walls.

   Fresh, **green oat** (*Avena sativa*) seeds have been
used as a mild antispasmodic and as a nourishing

nerve tonic for nervous prostration and exhaustion.
It is also helpful for overcoming the debilitating habit
of opium (morphine) use. Tests with the extract
show its antagonism to morphine. Studies also
indicate it has neither a stimulant nor a depressant
effect on the central nervous system.

This combination should be used three times
daily. It does not produce immediate, drug-like,
stimulant effects. The influence increases with
prolonged usage and the effects are more subtle than
the easily perceived surge derived from caffeine.
These herbs provide a fine-tuning of metabolic
activity in the physiological response to demands, not
a nerve-tingling, roller-coaster, joy ride.

Add one of the following formulas if needed.

Heart Tonic Formula

In cases in which diminished circulation to the
brain is the primary problem, additional herbs that
improve the function of the heart and help increase
blood vessel dilation can further help. Conditions
with poor mental functions due to reduced circulation are more commonly found in elderly individuals.

Balanced Blood Formula

Though controlling cholesterol levels in the
blood will not immediately improve mental function,
in the long run lowering blood lipids can help prevent deposits in blood vessels to the brain. Such
deposits may eventually diminish blood flow to the
brain and can serve as sites for clot formation that
may lead to strokes.

Soothing Sleep and Sedative Formula

Common complaints of our day are related to the
excessive mental and emotional demands of organiz-

ing time commitments, fulfilling multiple role obliga-
tions, and avoiding threats to personal security. The
tension this creates is improved through taking the
time to unwind mentally, emotionally, and physically.
Rest must be incorporated into the daily routine if
balance is to be maintained. Being alone, relaxing the
body, closing the eyes, and detaching the mind from
its cares helps immensely to relieve strain. At times
there is no opportunity to isolate oneself from the
sources of problems. If constant pressure, worry, or
experiences of terror result in insomnia, it may be
necessary to use a sleep aid to give the mind its
needed rest. Addictive and toxic medicines or drugs
only complicate the difficulties. Using a non-habit
forming, safe herbal sedative is a gentle way to help
get to sleep at bedtime. An herbal sedative does not
remove the problems, but it can help reduce the
difficulty of living with them.

    Valerian (*Valeriana officinalis*) root has a history
of use for sleeplessness and various spastic nervous
conditions. Aqueous extracts have been shown to
improve sleep quality. The essential oil components
of valerian including valeranone, valerenal, and
valerenic acid are sedative in their effects. The roots
have a peculiar odor derived from valepotriates which
are antispasmodic and tranquilizing. These
valepotriates decrease restlessness, anxiety, and
aggressiveness through their central nervous sedative
activity. Valepotriates also aid relaxation through
regulating autonomic nervous function. Unlike other
sedatives, valepotriates do not increase the toxicity of
alcohol but rather antagonize its effects. Valtrate, a
major valepotriate component, produces notable
changes in EEG (electroencephalogram) patterns and
reduces movement in the user. The valepotriates also
increase circulation to the heart.

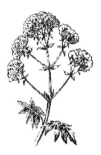

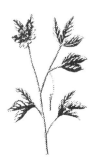

Passion flower (*Passiflora incarnata*) leaves are sedative and antispasmodic. They have been used for conditions of nervous irritability such as insomnia and restlessness. The leaves contain alkaloids (harman, harmine, and harmol) that reduce the breakdown of amine transmitter substances and flavonoids (vitexin, isovitexin, orientin, and isoorientin) that produce sedative effects. Vitexin antagonizes the amine transmitters and acts as an antispasmodic and anti-inflammatory agent. It also lowers blood pressure. Another component called maltol also produces sedative and relaxing effects.

Hops (*Humulus lupulus*) flower cones are another herbal remedy for sleeplessness. They have antispasmodic, anti-inflammatory, and sedative properties. The sedative activity is due to 2-methyl-3-buten-2-ol, a breakdown product of the humulones and lupulones in hops. This compound promotes sleep by its central nervous system depressant activity.

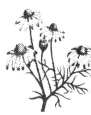

Chamomile (*Anthemis nobilis,* also called *Chamaemelum nobile*) flowers have a mild relaxant effect. This makes it a favorite herb for digestive problems and childhood upsets. The antispasmodic activity of chamomile is due to the flavonoid luteolin. Glycosides of luteolin and apigenin aid relaxation. Aromatic components of this fragrant herb include angelic acid esters, pinocarvone, and terpene hydrocarbons. The volatile compounds azulene and chamazulene are anti-inflammatory in their effects.

Anise (*Pimpinella anisum*) seeds are used both as an antispasmodic and for insomnia. The seeds are high in choline and contain the cholinergic transmitter compound. The oil of anise seeds is high in anethole which has estrogen effects that influence reproductive functions.

At times a sedative can be helpful even when

sleep is not the goal. When anxiety or nervousness interfere with purposeful activity, using small amounts of this formula for its calming and relaxing effects can be beneficial. In such cases it is taken in the low end of its dosage range from 1 to 5 times daily.

Add one of the following formulas if needed.

Bitter Digestive Tonic Formula

If anxiety interferes with the relaxation necessary to adequately digest a meal, then using a herbal digestive aid may help to avoid dyspepsia. Bitters together with calmative herbs provide the means for proper digestion.

Analgesic and Antispasmodic Formula

Pain and spasm can often be reduced by a calm state of mind. The aggravation caused by pain can also disturb ones serenity. A mild sedative helps to detach the mind from constant attention to a distracting painful condition. Muscular relaxation also helps to calm the mind and ease discomfort.

Phytoestrogen Aid Formula

Emotional swings can be a problem for some women during their climacteric. The experience of hormonal changes during these times increases the susceptibility to stress or aggravations. Selective use of a herbal sedative can ease the transition through some of the more trying moments at the age when menstrual cycles become irregular and finally cease.

Children's Calming Elixir Formula

Childhood is normally a time of high energy and activity. However, signs of chronic uncontrollable behavior suggests the possibility of such things as insecurity with parental relationships or an unsuitable home environment. Allergies or sensitivities to particular foods or food additives can be other underlying causes of emotional outbursts. If these reactions occur with frequency they should not be addressed simply by masking the symptoms with drugs. When occasional distress or discomfort produces anxiety in a child, it can usually be managed by using herbs that are calming. Irritability from teething or colic in an infant can be very disruptive, and the suffering child deserves relief for these physical problems. Many times anxiety will cause a stomachache or bad dreams in children, and they need comfort as well. The pleasant flavor of these carminative herbs that have calming properties makes them acceptable to children. In cases of fever where there is restlessness and the skin is dry, herbs that have diaphoretic activity can effectively increase sweating when taken in warm water or as a herbal tea. This helps the child to relax and cools the fever.

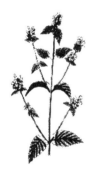

Catnip (*Nepeta cataria*) herb is a mild nervine for calming restlessness and irritability. It acts as a carminative for upset stomach and colic. It is used to relieve pain caused by spasms. Its warm extract is taken for its relaxing diaphoretic activity. The iridoid terpene nepetalactone is the attractive principle for cats from the oil of this plant. It is converted to nepetalic acid. Chemically similar compounds are present in the leaves and tops. Catnip oil, nepetalactone, and nepetalic acid from catnip have been shown to produce sedative effects in animals other than cats.

Chamomile (*Anthemis nobilis,* also called *Chamacmelum nobile*) flowers have frequently been used as a nervine for childhood ailments such as colic, upset stomach, fever, and restlessness. Chamomile has a relaxing effect on spasms, especially those of the stomach and intestines. Besides the carminative activity of its aromatic oil, the flavonoids in the flowers also have antispasmodic effects. The flavonoids include luteolin and the glycosides of apigenin and luteolin. These flavonoids and the aromatic components azulene and chamazulene have demonstrated anti-inflammatory activity as well.

Lemon balm (*Melissa officinalis*) herb is another antispasmodic carminative that produces diaphoretic effects when the extract is taken as a warm beverage. Besides relieving cramps it has been used as a nervine for anxiety. Its alcoholic distillate, aromatic oil, and terpene components all have sedative activity. The aromatic oil is antifungal and antibacterial, while its terpenes are antibacterial and antispasmodic. Lemon balm and its caffeic acid and rosmarinic acid constituents have shown antiviral effects. It contains the triterpene ursolic acid which is antibacterial and anti-inflammatory. Its flavonoid component luteolin glycoside is also anti-inflammatory.

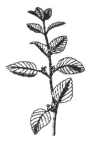

Peppermint (*Mentha piperita*) leaves are among the most well known carminatives for the relief of digestive upsets. The antispasmodic activity is present in the alcoholic extract. It is due mostly to the terpenes in the aromatic oil, especially menthol. The leaves are also mildly antiseptic due to their aromatic oil and ursolic acid content. In addition, the leaves contain flavonoids and rosmarinic acid and show some antiviral activity.

Hyssop (*Hyssopus officinalis)* flowers are used to relieve inflammations in the throat and intestines. Hyssop is both an expectorant and a carminative. For upper respiratory infections with mucus discharges and for gas and other digestive problems, the aromatic oil is an important component. The oil was shown to be active against both worms and tubercu-

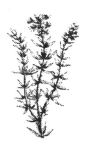

losis bacteria. Hyssop also contains a number of similar flavonoid glycosides and the antibacterial ursolic acid. Hyssop extracts have limited antiviral activity.

Elder (*Sambucus nigra*) flowers are used mostly as a diaphoretic to increase sweating when taken as a hot beverage. This may be due in part to their choline content. The extract is also used to relieve aching muscles. Elder flowers contain the flavonoids quercetol, kaempferol, and rutin. These flavonoids have anti-inflammatory effects. Kaempferol is also antispasmodic. The flowers contain the anti-inflammatory triterpenoid ursolic acid.

The sweetness given to this formula by glycerin helps to insure that children will take it willingly. It should be taken in warm water to increase both its relaxant and diaphoretic effects. Since it contains only mildly sedative herbs it can be used without fear of being too depressant for children.

Add the following formula if needed.

Antiviral and Antibacterial Formula

In cases of colds or the flu in children when greater rest and relaxation would aid in recovery, a calmative agent has its place. The infection can simultaneously be treated with simple herbal remedies that can help speed recovery.

INFLUENCES ON NERVOUS SYSTEM FUNCTIONS

MENTAL/EMOTIONAL OVERLOAD

Mind	Mood	Body
Stress	Anxiety	Tenseness
Restlessness	Irritability	
Insomnia	Anger	
Nightmares	Jealousy	

CALMING INFLUENCES

Physiologic	Somatic	Mental	Herbal
Calcium	Relaxation	Love	Siberian Ginseng
Magnesium	Slow Breathing	Forgiveness	Green Oats
Vitamin B	Warm Bath	Peaceful	Valerian
Complex	Sweating	Images	Passion Flower
Tryptophan	Quietude		Hops
	Darkness		Chamomile
	Strolling		Anise
			Catnip
			Lemon Balm
			Peppermint
			Hyssop
			Elder Flowers

MENTAL/EMOTIONAL DULLNESS

Mind	Mood	Body
Poor Attention	Insecurity	Sluggishness
Forgetfulness	Worry	
Indifference	Depression	

ALERTNESS ENHANCERS

Physiologic	Somatic	Mental	Herbal
Tyrosine	Inversion	Faith	Ginkgo
	Vigorous Exercise	Hope	Siberian Ginseng
	Rapid Breathing	Excitement	Gotu Kola
	Cold Water	Uplifting	Green Oats
	Up-tempo Music	Memories	
	Brisk Walking		

VII

WOMEN & MEN

Ovaries And Uterus

The events of a menstrual cycle are determined mainly by complex hormonal interactions. When hormonal imbalances occur, symptoms commonly arise prior to menstruation. Specific dietary adjustments and supplementation help to keep the reproductive system in women functioning normally.

The menstrual cycle in women is a process involving a complex interplay of factors. It chiefly involves rhythmic fluctuations of hormone levels. However, hormone release is affected by mental, emotional, and physical influences. Physical factors that interfere include travel, activity, exposure to light, temperature, humidity, odors, and food. The response of reproductive organs to hormones also depends on a woman's nutritional status. It is important to realize that great individual variability exists among women for the occurrence of the cycle and its phases. Since these differences can be entirely normal, the time periods mentioned below should only be regarded as average. Menarche is the time of the first menstrual period. It usually occurs between age nine and sixteen. Menstruation then reoccurs on a regular basis about once per month throughout a woman's life. The menstrual cycles are interrupted by pregnancies, after which their resumption is postponed by regular nursing. They continue through the climacteric. This is a time after age 40 when menstruation becomes diminished and irregular. They finally cease at menopause around age 50.

A typical menstrual cycle must be examined to appreciate the basic hormone changes and organ responses. **The cycle depends on three sources of endocrine hormones: the hypothalamus of the brain, the pituitary gland just below the hypothalamus, and the ovaries.** The hypothalamus secretes substances that cause the pituitary to release hormones which activate the ovaries. During the menstrual period the blood levels of the follicle stimulating hormone (FSH) begin to rise slightly. **After the period the pituitary FSH rise causes the production of estrogen by the ovary follicle to steadily increase.** Estrogen secretion causes a gradual increase in the production of cervical mucus that moistens the vagina. The follicular, or proliferation, phase is mainly characterized by thickening of the inner lining of the uterus. **The estrogen level eventually reaches a peak to which the hypothalamus responds.** The sensitivity of the hypothalamus to this peak can be influenced by sickness and physical or emotional stresses. The hypothalamus causes the pituitary to release a surge of FSH and luteinizing hormone (LH). **The pituitary LH surge stimulates the release of an egg by the ovary follicle, a process known as ovulation.** Just prior to ovulation the cervical mucus at the vaginal opening becomes slippery and/or stretchy. This first part of the cycle from the beginning of the period to ovulation is the most variable. It usually takes from one to three weeks.

At ovulation LH from the pituitary causes the ovarian follicle to begin changing. It grows into the corpus luteum (yellow body), and the luteal, or secretory, phase begins. **Estrogen output diminishes during the first week after ovulation, while progesterone production by the corpus luteum from the ovary increases rapidly.** Then together they peak one week after ovulation. The progesterone rise prepares the uterine lining for possible implantation of a fertilized egg. Progesterone also causes observable changes. It reduces vaginal secretions, stimulates the glands of the breasts, and raises the basal body temperature (taken before rising in the morning) after ovulation about 0.6°. **If no fertilized egg is implanted within one week after ovulation, estrogen and progesterone both decline during the second week.** This decline occurs as the LH drops and the corpus luteum degenerates. The uterine lining begins to deteriorate as the ovarian hormone levels fall. **Menstrual bleeding then occurs as the uterine lining is shed and expelled.** The bleeding period usually lasts for three to five days. The second part of the cycle from ovulation to the beginning of the period is usually quite regular and takes about two weeks. During menstruation the ovarian hormones reach low levels which stimulates the hypothalamus to begin a new cycle.

Estrogen helps to regulate the cycle by activating the hypothalamus with its drop just prior to the menstrual period and with its peak prior to ovulation. It also acts on the vaginal lining, the ducts in the breasts, the fallopian tubes, and uterine muscle. **Excessive estrogen (hyperestrogenism) can stimulate pituitary prolactin secretion and cause nausea, fluid retention, breast tenderness, depression, and longer periods.** Conditions correlated with hyperestrogenism include cystic breasts, cystic ovaries, uterine fibroids, and functional uterine bleeding due to proliferation of the uterine lining.   Factors that influence estrogen levels can disrupt the cycle and affect fertility. For instance, estrogen is converted to a less active form by the liver. If poor liver function slows this deactivation, stronger estrogen effects result. Obesity can lead to an increased conversion of other steroids to estrogen. Stress can increase adrenal production of estrogens and stimulate prolactin secretion.

Symptoms that occur before some women's periods are frequently related to hyperestrogenism. These symptoms include weight gain, edema, breast fullness, cramping, irritability, and depression. Combinations of these symptoms are collectively known as premenstrual syndrome (PMS). Carbohydrate craving, acne, headache, constipation, fatigue, and insomnia are also associated with PMS. Low progesterone can lead to symptoms similar to those from high estrogen levels. Prolactin stimulates milk production by the breasts after birth but may also be involved in PMS symptoms. Thyroid hormone is antagonistic to estrogen, so poor thyroid function can aggravate problems that are caused by estrogen. Reducing estrogen and prolactin effects and raising progesterone output may be the keys to reducing premenstrual symptoms. Lowering body weight and stress while improving liver and thyroid function are important considerations in resolving this condition.

Certain dietary practices help normalize the hormonal activity when applied regularly. Providing adequate iodine intake for thyroid activity is necessary. Avoiding daily consumption of goiter-causing raw vegetables from the cabbage family (cabbage, broccoli, Brussels sprouts, kale, cauliflower, rutabagas, and turnips) improves thyroid output. Eliminating caffeine, fat, sugar, and white flour in the diet and increasing consumption of complex carbohydrates (grains, beans, and starchy vegetables) is important. These changes help maintain blood sugar and energy balance, lower body weight, and reduce the metabolic demands on the liver. The increased intake of fiber from eating whole foods prevents constipation and improves excretion of estrogen by adsorption.

Taking supplements can be important for relieving premenstrual symptoms. Black currant oil and evening primrose oil supply GLA, a precursor of prostaglandins that counteract prolactin. Vitamin B_6 affects nerve transmitter substances that inhibit prolactin secretion and control mood swings. Vitamin B_6 also improves liver metabolism of estrogen and reduces water retention. The entire vitamin B complex aids in energy metabolism and stress management. Vitamin C is important in stress and improves mineral absorption. Calcium and magnesium alleviate cramping and nervous irritability and aid sleep. (Herbs that reduce uterine pain and cramping during the menstrual period are discussed under the Analgesic and Antispasmodic Formula for muscles.

Premenstrual Ease Formula

Certain conditions seem to make women more susceptible to PMS symptoms. After giving birth or after stopping birth control pills, hormonal imbalance is typical as the cycles readjust. High stress, poor diet, frequent weight gain and loss, aging, conflicts in relationships, recreational drugs, and medications can all interfere with the regulation of hormonal changes. In addition to dietary changes, adequate exercise and rest may be the most important means of helping the body to regain control of the fluctuations. At times it may become necessary to employ other support, such as the following herbs, to prevent symptoms from becoming debilitating.

Chaste tree (*Vitex agnus-castus*) berries have been recognized as having hormonal effects that help restore menstrual period regularity. These have also been used for irritability and depression associated with reproductive functions. The berries are believed to act on the hypothalamus to cause the pituitary to release LH. This stimulates corpus luteum secretions after ovulation occurs. Ultimately, a progesterone-like effect is produced which has been demonstrated in animals. Chaste tree alcoholic extract also inhibits prolactin secretion by pitutitary cells. Symptomatic improvement of premenstrual water retention and acne have been documented. The berries and seeds contain casticin as their major flavonoid and other minor flavonols as well. The berries also contain an aromatic oil with antibacterial terpenes.

Wild Yam (*Dioscorea villosa*) root is antispasmodic. It has been used for bilious colic and painful uterine contractions. Wild yam has also been taken to allay nausea due to high hormone levels. The root contains a steroidal sapogenin called diosgenin. Since diosgenin has only slight anticonvulsant effects, other components must be responsible for the antispasmodic activity. Diosgenin is used commercially to synthesize progesterone. However, when given orally to animals it has an estrogenic effect about 1/10 that of synthetic estrogen. Diosgenin can therefore compete with estrogen for receptor sites and thereby reduce the overall estrogen effect.

Dong quai (*Angelica sinensis*, also known as *A. polymorpha* var. *sinensis*) root has long been popular in China for regulating the menstrual cycle and helping to make the period less painful. It is used for its antispasmodic, analgesic, sedative, and anti-inflammatory properties. It was also found to reduce the production of IgE antibodies. Ferulic acid, one of its active components, reduces uterine contractions and heart arrhythmias. The root extract, ferulic acid, and ligustilide, a major phthalide component of dong quai root aromatic oil, all inhibit platelet clumping necessary for clotting. For this reason dong quai should not be used after menstrual bleeding has started. Ligustilide is a uterine antispasmodic. It and other phthalide components are also antispasmodic for air passages of the lungs.

Blue cohosh (*Caulophyllum thalictroides*) root was originally used by American Indians to aid in childbirth. It has since been utilized to regulate suppressed menstrual flow. As a diuretic it was taken to reduce water retention. Blue cohosh also was used for breast and pelvic pain dependant on congestion. While blue cohosh root acts to tone the uterus, it has the effect of relaxing muscles that are in spasm. This is due to its alkaloid methylcytisine. The uterine tonic effect is due to saponins that have hederagenin as the aglycone.

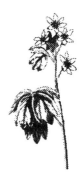

This herbal combination is intended for use during the luteal phase of the cycle. The use of these herbs should begin when the signs of ovulation have been observed and should end when the period starts. The usual dose of 15-30 drops may be taken 1-5 times daily according to need. For this condition as for others, better results can be expected if additional supportive measures are utilized.

Add one of the following formulas if needed.

Liver Tonic Formula

Since the liver plays such an important role in the metabolism of estrogen, its proper function is essential for the appropriate hormonal balance to be maintained. By supporting the liver's metabolic and excretory activities the accumulation of potent steroidal hormones is less likely.

Analgesic and Antispasmodic Formula

Intestinal or pelvic discomfort and uterine spasm are sometimes associated with premenstrual tension. Temporary relief can be provided by agents used for muscular pain. These antispasmodic herbs have commonly been used to treat menstrual disorders. It may be helpful to continue using them during the period if discomfort persists.

Phytoestrogen Aid Formula

When phytoestrogens bind to estrogen receptors their effect is less than that of ovarian estrogens would be. Therefore the mild effects of herbs help to reduce the strong effects of estrogen by competing for estrogen receptor sites. This is beneficial for symptoms associated with high estrogen levels. The herbs for other premenstrual symptoms can also be of benefit during menopause when these same conditions occur.

Phytoestrogen Aid Formula

Menopause is another time of adjustment to hormonal changes that proves difficult for many women. As ovarian hormone concentrations drop, symptoms commonly seen include hot flashes, headaches, irritability, depression, fatigue, and insomnia. Physical changes after menopause include vaginal thinning and dryness and reduction of calcium in the bones. The calcium loss should be addressed by supplementing calcium and a source of vitamin D such as cod liver oil. Some of these changes can be treated symptomatically with herbs. Another means of aiding the process is by supplying an external source of estrogen. These plants contain components with mild estrogen activity and should help to reduce the intensity of the symptoms. These low potency phytoestrogens include sterols, coumestans, and isoflavones. High doses may be necessary to provide sufficient relief in some cases.

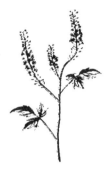

Black cohosh (*Cimicifuga racemosa*) root is a sedative and antispasmodic. It is known for its effect on the uterus which helps bring on the period. It is also commonly taken for menopausal symptoms. The use of black cohosh for this condition is mainly due to the root's estrogenic activity. This activity was shown by root extracts increasing the weight of ovaries and uteri and the number of corpora lutea in juvenile animals. The root contains at least three different estrogenic compounds, one of which is the isoflavone formononetin. Though formononetin had no effect on the LH, the extract of black cohosh reduced pituitary LH output. Excessive amounts of black cohosh can cause headache and/or nausea.

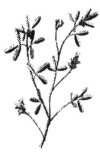

The **alfalfa** (*Medicago sativa*) plant is generally thought of as a digestive tonic for humans. However, it also contains many nonsteroid phytoestrogens. The most abundant and most potent of these is the coumestan called coumestrol. The isoflavone components listed in order according to their concentration in alfalfa are formononetin, biochanin A, daidzein, and genistein. This order is the reverse of their comparative estrogenic potencies. When estrogen is present these phytoestrogens compete with it for binding to estrogen receptors. The phytoestrogens produce some estrogenic activity, but they reduce the effect that estrogen by itself would have. Except for formononetin, this competition also occurs at receptors on cancerous human breast cells where both estrogen and phytoestrogens stimulated growth. In addition to phytoestrogens alfalfa also contains a substance that inhibits pituitary LH.

Hops (*Humulus lupulus*) flower cones are calming and sedative. They have traditionally been used for restlessness and insomnia. The diuretic effect of hops is used in cases of water retention. Hops also acts as a uterine sedative and relieves menstrual cramps, especially if taken prior to their onset. Some studies have shown hops to have phytoestrogen activity, and estradiol (a strong estrogenic steroid) was identified in a fat-soluble extract of hops. Other studies on hops estrogen activity refute these findings. Several other substances that inhibit progesterone production have been discovered in hops.

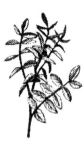

Licorice (*Glycyrrhiza glabra*) root does not have a long history of use for conditions specifically associated with women. However, its extract was found to have an estrogenic effect in animals. Licorice root contains estriol (a mild estrogen steroid), the isoflavone formononetin, and the coumestans glycyrol, isoglycyrol, and methylglycyrol. In very large amounts the component glycyrrhizin inhibits estrogen. The amount of licorice in combinations is kept small, since the fluid retention and potassium loss caused glycyrrhizin prohibits the use of large doses over an extended period of time. It should not be used in cases of high blood pressure or heart disease.

Anise (*Pimpinella anisum*) oil extracted from the seeds has a flavor like that of licorice. It has also shown estrogenic activity. However, in the case of anise it is due to polymers of the aromatic oil component anethole. Anise seed has been used to promote the onset of menstruation and improve milk production in nursing mothers. It is also a pleasant tasting carminative which relieves nausea and gas and alleviates gastrointestinal cramps.

Motherwort (*Leonurus cardiaca*) flowering tops

are renowned for allaying the trials of menopause. Motherwort is used to calm nervous tension and irritability and to relieve insomnia in women. The alcoholic extract was shown in several studies to have antispasmodic and sedative properties. It also lowers blood pressure. These effects have not been correlated with specific components. Motherwort contains the alkaloid leonurine, sterols, flavonoid glycosides, and many iridoid glycosides including leonuride, ajugoside, and galiridoside.

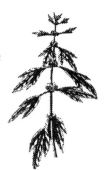

Though phytoestrogens bind to estrogen receptors in the body their effect is not as potent as ovarian estrogens. Therefore, if they are used at a younger age during the menstrual cycle, they compete with the body's own estrogen for receptor sites. This can actually reduce the ovarian estrogen's activity. Some phytoestrogens also act on the hypothalamus and reduce the output of the pituitary hormones that stimulate the ovaries. Still other nonestrogenic compounds inhibit the output or effects of pituitary LH. This can result in less estrogen production by the ovaries. To inhibit the effects of hyperestrogenism the herbs should be taken from one week after ovulation and until the start of the menstrual period about one week later. For this effect the dose should be kept low. Thus, phytoestrogens can produce estrogen effects after menopause or reduce excessive estrogen activity prior to the climacteric. The result depends upon the dose and whether significant amounts of estrogen are already present in the body or not.

Add one of the following formulas if needed.

Premenstrual Ease Formula

If excessive estrogen is a probable cause of premenstrual symptoms, then using low potency phytoestrogens in small amounts can reduce the estrogen effect by competing for receptor sites. The use of phytoestrogens in this way does not address the root problems, but may help to relieve unpleasant symptoms until the normal hormonal balance is achieved through other methods such as using the appropriate premenstrual herbs.

Soothing Sleep and Sedative Formula

When addressing the symptoms associated with menopause, the use of phytoestrogens may not completely alleviate some of the symptoms. If insomnia remains a disruptive complication, then herbs that help relax the body and calm the mind will work to great advantage.

HORMONAL BALANCE IN WOMEN

ESTROGEN EXCESS

Signs and Symptoms	Causes and Aggravations	Use Estrogen Inhibition
Nausea	Poor Liver Function	Phytoestrogens
Fluid Retention	Obesity	(small doses):
Breast Tenderness	Stress	Wild Yam
Depression	Prolactin Secretion	Black Cohosh
Long Periods	Low Progesterone	Alfalfa
Cystic Breasts	Low Thyroid Function	Hops
Cystic Ovaries		Licorice
Uterine Fibroids		Anise
Uterine Bleeding		

OTHER MEANS FOR REDUCING ESTROGEN EFFECTS

Supporting The Liver

Eliminate Caffeine
Increase Fiber In Diet
Increase Elimination
Vitamin B6
Avoid Drugs

Counteracting Prolactin

Black Currant Oil
Evening Primrose Oil
Vitamin B6

Losing Weight

Decrease Fat In Diet
Decrease Sugar, White Flour
Increase Complex Carbohydrates

Promoting Progesterone

Chaste Tree Berries

Buffering Stress

Vitamin B Complex
Vitamin C
Calcium
Magnesium

Supporting The Thyroid

Provide Iodide In Diet
Avoid Daily Raw Cruciferae:
Cabbage
Broccoli
Cauliflower
Rutabagas
Turnips

ADDITIONAL RELIEF FOR PMS SYMPTOMS

Water Retention	Uterine Cramps	Irritability	Insomnia	Nausea	Acne
Chaste Tree	Dong Quai	Dong Quai	Motherwort	Wild Yam	Chaste Tree
Blue Cohosh	Wild Yam	Motherwort	Hops	Anise	
Hops	Blue Cohosh	Black Cohosh	Calcium		
Vitamin B$_6$	Black Cohosh	Hops	Magnesium		
	Hops	Calcium			
	Calcium	Magnesium			
	Magnesium				

ESTROGEN INSUFFICIENCY

Signs & Symptoms	Use Estrogen Support
Hot Flashes	Phytoestrogens
Headaches	(larger doses):
Irritability	Black Cohosh
Depression	Alfalfa
Fatigue	Hops
Insomnia	Anise
Vaginal Dryness	Licorice
Bone Calcium Loss	

ADDITIONAL RELIEF FOR MENOPAUSAL SYMPTOMS

Irritability	Insomnia	Bone Weakening
Motherwort	Motherwort	Calcium
Black Cohosh	Hops	Vitamin D
Hops		Cod Liver Oil

Testes And Prostate

While the testes are the source of testosterone and sperm, the prostate is associated with these and supplies additional secretions to the semen. The prostate becomes problematic when it is enlarged or inflamed.

The secretion of the male hormone testosterone and the production of sperm by the testes is controlled through the release of the pituitary hormones. Though the levels of these hormones vary over time, they do not have the estreme cyclic fluctuations that occur in women. Since the pituitary is regulated by the hypothalamus of the brain, mental/emotional states do influence the release of these gonadotropins somewhat.

Testosterone secretion by the testes is stimulated by LH release from the pituitary. The feedback effect of testosterone on the hypothalamus inhibits the signal for pituitary release of LH. Puberty begins in boys around the age of ten when this hypothalamic sensitivity diminishes. This initiates pituitary LH signals to increase testosterone production, resulting in a number of changes in the body. These include a progressive enlargement of the testes and the prostate until about the age of 20. Testosterone production peaks at age 20 and then begins a gradual decline. It drops significantly around age 50 at which time sexual function usually diminishes also. Symptoms of this climacteric in men are not as common or severe as they are in women. Hot flashes, a sense of suffocation, or mental/emotional symptoms occasionally occur. Testosterone secretion and sperm production continue at a low level until death.

Sperm develop under the influence of pituitary FSH and testosterone. The inability to produce sperm after puberty may be permanent due to a number of chromosomal, traumatic, toxic, or infectious causes that cause the testes to atrophy. It can be temporarily caused by pituitary disorders or the chronic use of drugs including marijuana and corticosteroids. Another possible cause is the regular exposure of the testicles to high temperatures such as in prolonged fever. The failure of the testes to descend into the scrotum prior to puberty can result in permanent infertility due to their continual exposure to the warmer interior of the body. Long soaks in a hot tub taken daily or wearing snug jockey shorts regularly can lead to a temporary block in sperm production. The blood engorgement around the testes from a varicocele raises the temperature in a similar fashion.

The prostate is analogous to the female uterus and surrounds the upper urethra just below the bladder. It is one of the organs of the body that is most affected by testosterone. Cancer of the prostate causes 2-3% of deaths in men, and it is stimulated by testosterone. (Castration has been used to prevent testosterone production as a means of treating prostatic cancer.) The prostate converts testosterone to dihydrotestosterone. Dihydrotestosterone is bound to receptors of prostate cells and then to the nuclei of these cells. This causes increased DNA replication and protein production which enlarges the gland. **When it contracts the prostate contributes a thin, milky, alkaline fluid to the semen.** After age 20 it retains a fairly stationary size until around 40 to 50 years of age. Then it begins to degenerate in some men as testosterone levels fall. A benign enlargement of the prostate often occurs after age 50 which narrows the urethra and causes urinary obstruction.

If there is tenderness in the area of the prostate or if blood is noticed in the urine, it is important to be examined by a doctor to check for prostate infection or cancer. Cases of acute infection or cancer of the prostate require medical intervention. **A number of substances and methods can be used to help control chronic prostate inflammation or benign enlargement.** The consumption of certain pumpkin seeds (*Cucurbita pepo* var. *styriaca*) has been found to be helpful. Supplements of vitamins A and C and the mineral zinc are also beneficial. Local massage of the prostate is helpful in cases of chronic, but not acute, inflammation. If constipation is involved, more fluid and fiber must be included in the diet in the form of fresh fruit and vegetables. Prolonged sitting or standing should be avoided. Regular walking and exercise help stimulate circulation to the pelvis. A specific exercise for this area (called Kegel's exercises) is to contract the muscles of the pelvic area (between the rectum and the bladder) and hold the contraction for a few seconds. This helps to keep the muscles of this region in tone.

An important method to improve pelvic circulation in men or women is the practice of alternating sitz baths. This is done by using a tub with hot water and another with cold water. Horsetail or chamomile tea can be added to the hot water. Begin by sitting with just the hips, buttocks, and lower abdomen in the hot tub for 2-5 minutes. The hot water should come about one inch above the navel. The heat relaxes the tissues and blood vessels which brings in more nutrients and fresh blood to the region. Then

get out and immediately sit in the cold tub for 20 to
60 seconds. The cold water level should be about one
inch below the navel. The cold contracts the tissues
and vessels which moves out the blood with its waste
and prevents congestion. Repeat this cycle several
times and always end with the cold water. When
finished drying off, cover up and lie down to rest for
a short while. These sitz baths can be repeated two
or three times per week. They should not be done if
there is an acute infection of the genitourinary tract.

Prostate Tonic Formula

The bladder outlet obstruction caused by prostate
enlargement is due to growth of its glandular nodules. As the obstruction progresses the symptoms of
urinary frequency, urgency, and nighttime urination
become worse. Decreased size and force of the
urinary stream develop, and dribbling is common.
The retention of urine can lead to chronic secondary
infections of the bladder and prostate. It can also
result in stone formation in the bladder. Alcohol,
anesthetics, and drugs that have adrenergic or anti-
cholinergic effects can cause a complete, sudden
blockage of the genitourinary tract. If the retention is
prolonged, it may result in kidney damage and
failure. It is important to intervene before the
symptoms progress too far. Since resolving the
condition nonsurgically is a slow process, it is necessary to simultaneously reduce congestion and control
infections. The herbal approach to nonmalignant
prostate enlargements is best used early in the course
of the condition to relieve symptoms and prevent
kidney involvement.

Saw palmetto (*Serenoa serrulata,* also called *S.
repens*) berries have been used as a tonic for pelvic
organs, especially for the enlarged prostate in elderly

men. An extract of the berries has been shown to
reduce edema. This extract also slightly inhibits
conversion of testosterone to a more active compound, reduces the binding of both hormonal compounds to their receptors in human cells, and reduces
the hormonal receptors in the nuclei of human
prostate cells. In placebo-controlled studies it was
shown to significantly improve the symptoms of
benign prostate enlargement. Fatty alcohols and high
molecular weight alcohol constituents from the
extract were shown to be active in reducing prostate
weight. Though sitosterol from the fruit can have
mild estrogenic activity if it is concentrated, the
extract actually functions as an antiestrogen. Other
alcohols, triterpenes, and sterols contribute to the
activity of the extract.

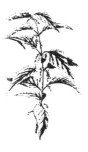

    Nettle (*Urtica dioica*) roots have also been used
to treat enlarged prostate. A clinical study showed
the root extract was helpful in relieving symptoms
due to prostate enlargement. The root contains
abundant sitosterol and other sterols and their glycosides. Nettle roots also contain isolectins that stimulate production of certain white blood cells that fight
infections.

    Pipsissewa (*Chimaphila umbellata*) leaves have
been used as a diuretic for kidney problems and
urinary discharges. It has been especially recommended for chronic irritation or inflammation of the
prostate. The leaves contain the phenolic glycoside
arbutin which is changed to hydroquinone in the
kidneys. The broad antibacterial activity of arbutin is
ascribed to this chemical transformation that occurs
in alkaline urine. The antiseptic activity can prevent
infections in cases of urinary retention.

    Narrow-leafed echinacea (*Echinacea angustifolia*)
root has been used for infections of the genitourinary

tract because of it immune-enhancing properties.
The isobutylamides, echinacoside, and cynarin in
echinacea increase phagocyte activity. When combined with saw palmetto and a chemical antispasmodic, echinacea was found to be helpful in cases of
prostatic inflammation and enlarged prostate. The oil
in echinacea root has antitumor activity.

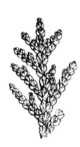

Yellow cedar (*Thuja occidentalis*) leaves contain a
high concentration of thujone in their aromatic oil.
They have been used to relieve dribbling urine due to
an enlarged prostate commonly found in elderly men.
The leaf extract has been shown to influence the first
phase of immune phagocytosis in a manner different
from echinacea. **Thujone is highly antiseptic and can
be toxic if taken in too large of a dosage.**

Ocotillo (*Fouquieria splendens*) bark has been
used to relieve conditions associated with pelvic
congestion. This is most likely due to its effect on the
liver. The bark contains the iridoid glycoside
adoxoside. The aglycone of adoxoside increases the
output of bile. The triterpenes ocotillol, fouquierol,
and isofouquierol found in the bark are metabolized
to dammarenediol which is stored in the root.
Dammarenediol and isofouquierol have shown
antiviral activity against herpes.

These herbs can be used to advantage in cases of
infection or inflammation of the prostate. Chronic
prostate inflammation is difficult to resolve, and
supportive approaches should also be applied. The
same is true of helping prostate enlargement in old
age. Herbs should not be used to the exclusion of
other substances and techniques. To control chronic
conditions it is important to use methods that contribute to the general health as well as to the improvement of the specific area of concern. Maintaining
activity in old age is a crucial aspect of maintaining

good health. This can be applied to mental, physical, and sexual functions.

Add the following formula if needed.

Diuretic and Urinary Antiseptic Formula

Bladder infections which commonly accompany enlargement of the prostate gland can be reduced through prevention or treatment with herbal antiseptic diuretics. Since urinary retention is one of the most frequent problems associated with prostate enlargement, the periodic presence in the urine of antiseptics that reduce bacterial growth is preferable to waiting to treat an established infection of the bladder or one that has reached the kidneys.

MALE GLANDULAR CONDITIONS

TESTICULAR INFERTILITY

Permanent Causes

Undescended Testes
Chromosome Defects
Orchitis
Testicular Trauma
Environmental Toxins

Reversible Causes

Pituitary Disorders
Chronic Marijuana Use
Chronic Corticosteroid Use
Prolonged Fever
Varicocele
Snug Jockey Shorts
Daily Pelvic Heat Exposure

PROSTATIC ENLARGEMENTS

Beneficial Additions to Diet

Vitamin A
Vitamin C
Zinc
Styriaca Pumpkin Seeds
Fluids and Fiber

Advantageous Routines

Walking
Kegel's Exercises
Alternating Sitz Baths
Regular Sexual Activity

HERBS FOR PROSTATIC ENLARGEMENTS

Chronic Prostatic Inflammation

Pipsissewa
Echinacea
Yellow Cedar
Ocotillo
Saw Palmetto

Benign Prostatic Hypertrophy

Saw Palmetto
Nettle Roots
Yellow Cedar
Ocotillo

VIII
ACHES & PAINS

Muscles And Joints

The advantages to be gained from physical activity are best achieved when exercise is regular and preparation, care, and moderation are practiced. Physiotherapy is a primary means of treating occupational, sports, or other musculoskeletal injuries. Local and internal remedies can further aid in recovery.

The benefits of exercise are many. It strengthens the heart and other muscles of the body. Circulation is improved by exercise, so more nutrients are delivered and waste is better removed from tissues. Exercise deepens breathing, so the diaphragm gives the abdominal organs a valuable massage. These ordinary benefits are lost for many since technology has done much to reduce physical activity in everyday work routines. Most Americans now enjoy the relative ease of life with automation. In times past the demands of everyday life required great exertion. This ranged from field work to grinding and kneading flour, pumping and carrying water, scrubbing laundry and sweeping floors, chopping and carrying wood, and walking almost everywhere. Physical labor is still important and necessary in our modern world. But for many, exercise is usually separated from work as a form of recreation. **Some sort of**

regular, vigorous physical activity is necessary for everyone.

While some people work or excerise to the point of causing stress injuries, others abuse their bodies by avoiding physical activity as much as possible. Especially dangerous is the sedentary fan who transforms into a dynamo known as the weekend warrior. Such long-lost competitors occasionally seek to impress friends or acquaintances with their former skills, but they are simply asking for trouble. **For a person who fails to maintain their conditioning, the gauge for recreational competition should be pleasure and not heroic success.** Even in these cases a little effort beforehand can provide important protection.

Before engaging in physically demanding activity a physical evaluation is in order. It is important to check the heart, circulation, reflexes, and joints. Poor alignment of bones creates strain on muscles and irritation at the joints, since both of these are involved in all movements. This most commonly occurs with the spine. The situation is compounded by the close proximity of emerging spinal nerves. Assessment and correction of bony malalignments by specialists in manipulation are important first steps in avoiding unnecessary pain and damage.

Preventing injury also involves determining what equipment and other protective measures are appropriate. Unnecessary stresses exerted on weight bearing joints of the spine, legs, and feet are especially important to avoid. For example, running on concrete in ordinary shoes produces a pounding of these joint surfaces. This can lead to acute or chronic inflammation, so appropriate footwear is an important consideration. Overweight individuals need to emphasize cycling or swimming in their routines to avoid undue trauma to weight bearing joints.

Participating safely in strenuous activities requires some prior physical preparation. This includes movement and stretching of the major muscle groups. Stretching in all directions helps to insure that when one muscle group is contracting its opposing group will not create too much resistance. The more muscular a person is, the more important stretching becomes to prevent straining or pulling tight muscles. This is a necessary part of every warm-up routine. **Maintaining balance in muscle strength can help prevent injury.** To promote this exercises that develop opposing muscle groups are important. Physical labor that increases muscle bulk also leads to greater tone. In this case regular stretching is needed to maintain flexibility and reduce injuries. After vigorous exercise muscles become more contracted than normal, so light movements that help them relax is a good way to cool down.

While steroid abuse occurs among some enthusiasts, most people who exercise are concerned with overall health and not just physical appearance. Many sports participants develop a knowledge of nutrition and the dangers of physical and chemical excesses. Those who train regularly to pursue long-term personal goals respond to the body's danger signals and avoid injury. Competitive athletics can be a different matter. Overzealous coaches or players may think that it is appropriate to sacrifice health for performance. **While athletes can suffer unnecessarily by taking unwarranted risks, the same is true of occupational hazards.** While workplaces and routines have been improved in many ways to make them safer, job-related injuries are still all too commonplace. The demands of productivity can takes precedence over health concerns for some when their burden of responsibility requires that they maintain their current livelihood.

Muscle spasms occur from overuse or as a result of chemical imbalances. When there is a tendency to develop cramps, calcium and magnesium supplements help to prevent them. Acute cramps are best given immediate relief by contracting the opposing muscle group against resistance. Massage passively stretches spastic muscles and helps them to relax. It also improves local circulation. Simple but effective massage can be done on oneself, especially on the feet. Back spasms tend to occur on one side. They impair both spinal flexibility and alignment. Spasms then develop on the opposite side to compensate which further complicates the problem. Spinal manipulation is usually necessary to correct the spinal fixations that occur with such conditions. Heat or hot baths provide a safe and effective means to relax muscle spasms that occur from overuse or inflammation. **Ointments and balms that contain herbal components are effective as topical analgesics and/or counterirritants for temporary relief muscle spasms or inflammations.** These compounds usually contain camphor, methyl salicylate (wintergreen oil), menthol (peppermint oil), eucalyptol (eucalyptus oil), cinnamaldehyde (cinnamon oil), and/or capsaicin (cayenne). Clinically, continuous stimulation of a spastic muscle with sinusoidal electrical current can fatigue it and cause it to relax.

Excessive repetitive activity or exercise unfailingly leads to irritation. For instance, the trauma from continual movement of a muscle tendon over an area can inflame the lubricating sheath and cause tendinitis or bursitis. **Resting the inflamed structure is necessary initially for it to begin healing.** Passive movements should be undertaken soon thereafter to avoid developing adhesions. Local ice massage for five to seven minutes until the skin becomes numb helps relieve the pain. **Relief for inflammation and recovery from soft tissue injuries can be speeded by taking proteolytic enzymes orally between meals prior to and after damage occurs.** These enzymes include bromelain from pineapple or papain from papaya. Most sudden athletic injuries involve muscle bruises and strains, sprained or torn joint ligaments, and subluxated, dislocated, or broken bones. Many of the same applications used for cramps can be applied to sprains and strains after the acute stage has passed. In the acute stage following trauma cold should be applied locally to reduce the pain, swelling, and internal bleeding. From 24-48 hours after an injury heat is used to increase the circulation and aid healing. Herbal extracts applied topically to aid the healing of injuries include those made from arnica and calendula flowers, comfrey root, St. Johnswort and witch hazel.

Many injuries and ailments that require clinical attention benefit from additional forms of physiotherapy besides rest, heat, and massage. For chronic conditions such as fibrositis (rheumatism) and arthritis, diathermy provides deep heating to increase circulation and healing. Ultrasonic treatment is very helpful for bringing local heating to structures on or near the surface of the bones. These high frequency sound waves also improve fluid movement and reduce local swelling that occurs with acute strain or sprain injuries or chronic inflammation. Pain due to circulatory impingement or nerve entrapment by spastic muscular nodules can be effectively relieved by galvanic, interferential, or other electrical currents. After the tissues are heated and spasms are relaxed manipulation of the spine or other joints can be of great benefit.

Analgesic and Antispasmodic Formula

Local physical treatments for soft tissue strain, inflammation, and spasm are by their nature short-term applications. The period between these treatments is intended to give time for healing, since the symptoms that continue to persist limit activity. While discomfort is an incentive to provide rest for the injured part, complete inactivity is not always possible or even desirable. The condition can become worse when lack of movement due to pain reduces local circulation. This can result in excessive fibrous tissue growth or adhesions. Even when activity needs to be restricted it is desirable to make the condition more bearable and to maintain some degree of function. Herbal agents to help control pain and relax muscles can be of benefit so long as their use does not result in overactivity and reinjury. These same herbs are also helpful to temporarily alleviate painful uterine cramping and pelvic discomfort during the menstrual period.

Kava kava (*Piper methysticum*) root is a sedative used in the South Pacific to allay anxiety and reduce fatigue. It has a central nervous system tranquilizing activity and an anesthetic effect on nerve pain. The root is also used to relax skeletal muscles and menstrual cramps. Kava kava contains a number of pyrones including kawain, methysticin, and yangonin and other less potent derivatives of these. These pyrones are anesthetic, anti-inflammatory, and antispasmodic. They reduce body temperature and spontaneous muscle movement. While kawain and its derivative produce their maximum anticonvulsive effect rapidly (after 10 min.) and for a short period (40-60 min.), methysticin and its derivative have a stronger anticonvulsive activity that is delayed (for 45-60 min.) and prolonged (2-4 hrs.). Yangonin's maximum effect is much less potent and even more delayed (2 hrs.). Yangonin and its derivative act synergistically with the other pyrones to lower body temperature, relax muscles and prevent convulsions.

Black cohosh (*Cimicifuga racemosa*, formerly called *Actea racemosa*) root is another herb that is used as a sedative for spasmodic conditions. While it has generally been applied to rheumatic pain of muscles and joints, it is frequently employed as a specific remedy for uterine pains with pelvic congestion and soreness. Tests showed the extract to have no sedative action on the brain, though it was a potent muscular relaxant for the uterus and intestines. Its pain-relieving effects are due in part to the salicylic acid content of the root. The root also contains the triterpene actein which increases peripheral blood flow.

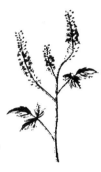

Jamaica dogwood (*Piscidia erythrina*) root bark has sedative, antispasmodic, and anti-inflammatory properties. It is used to control pain and relieve spasms, especially of the uterus. It has also been employed for nervousness and insomnia. The root bark has shown potent uterine sedative properties. Piscidone and di-isoprenyl-isoflavone are active isoflavones components that inhibit uterine contractions. Rotenone and the isoflavone ichthynone are bark components that act as potent fish toxins.

Ginger (*Zingiber officinale*) root is used to ease congestion and promote perspiration by stimulating the circulation. Its applications include painful intestinal spasms and the promotion of the menstrual flow in cases where it is suppressed. Ginger extract was shown to block spasms due to the activity of its gingerol and galanolactone. Patients having rheumatoid arthritis reported pain relief after consuming ginger for several months. This appears to be due in

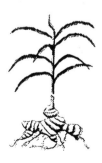

part to ginger blocking production of pro-inflamma-
tory thromboxanes. Its pungent gingerol,
gingerdione, and shogaol components inhibit the
enzymes that produce other inflammatory products
including 2-series prostaglandins and leukotrienes.
The combination of these anti-inflammatory and
antispasmodic effects suggest its usefulness for
migraine headaches.

Some of the herbs in this formula have potent
effects and require a lower dose than is used for other
formulas. Between 5 to 15 drops taken three times
each day is usually adequate to control pain and
spasm associated with soft tissue irritation or inflammation. In cases of injuries this formula would be
used after the fact, but for menstrual pain and cramping it would be most effective to take before the
discomfort becomes too severe.

Add one of the following formulas if needed.

Premenstrual Ease Formula

Menstrual cramps can be especially disturbing
when they follow a time of physical and emotional
disruption at the end of the menstrual cycle. The
severity of cramps during the menstrual period may
be perceived as less aggravating when premenstrual
symptoms are minimal. Herbs that help to maintain
a normal hormonal balance will thereby support
normal menstrual function as well.

Soothing Sleep and Sedative Formula

At times the relief of pain and muscular tension
demand greater rest and assisted relaxation. Mild
herbal calmatives not only relieve tension but also
alleviate the anxiety that exaggerates the perception of
discomfort.

Anti-Inflammatory Formula

Soft tissue pain is usually due to inflammation of the muscle fibers or connective tissue. Resolving the inflammation removes the cause of the pain. The discomfort of an inflamed joint can include local muscle spasms which reduce mobility by a splinting effect. While working to reduce the inflammation of joints or connective tissues, relieving the associated pain and muscular tension helps to make these condition more tolerable and improves the circulation to the area.

Anti-Inflammatory Formula

Chronic pain of the muscles, joints, and connective tissue associated with long-term trauma, metabolic or immune imbalance, and aging requires more than simply reducing nerve sensitivity to irritation. Inflammatory processes must be controlled if persistent relief is to be achieved. Though steroids like cortisone effectively block inflammation, they cannot be taken regularly or serious side effects will develop and destroy the general health. The side effects from steroid use of long duration include weakening of muscles and bones, heart failure, glaucoma, diabetes, headaches, and gastrointestinal ulceration. Effective doses of nonsteroidal anti-inflammatory medicines such as aspirin can cause stomach ulceration, renal disease, bronchospasm, ringing in the ears, and other symptoms that prevent their prolonged use. Herbs that reduce inflammation without causing significant side effects can help bring welcome relief to sufferers.

Devil's claw (*Harpagophytum procumbens*) grows in southern Africa. Its roots (tubers) have recently become popular in Europe for pain relief. In addition, their anti-inflammatory properties have led to their use for rheumatic complaints such as arthritis. The roots contain three main iridoids: harpagide, harpagoside, and procumbide. Root extracts and harpagoside were effective in tests that demonstrated their analgesic and anti-inflammatory effects. An extract and the harpagoside aglycone were effective against arthritis. Better results were obtained for semichronic than for acute inflammation. The extracts showed no toxicity, while the toxicity of pure harpagoside was low.

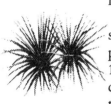

Yucca (*Yucca spp.*) roots are a rich source of steroidal saponins. Extracted saponins were tested as part of a clinical trial of arthritis therapies. Of the 149 patients with chronic arthritis studied in a double-blind trial, from one half to two thirds of those receiving the saponins reported favorable results including less pain, stiffness, and swelling. No reactions or toxicity were found either clinically or with lab tests. An anti-inflammatory yucca saponin extract was shown to contain the sapogenins (saponin aglycones) yuccagenin and kammogenin which are found in a number of species. Smilagenin and sarsasapogenin, the more common sapogenins in yucca species, can be chemically converted to a useful cortisone intermediate.

Black cohosh (*Cimicifuga racemosa,* formerly known as *Actea racemosa*) root is a remedy that has been used for a wide variety of rheumatic conditions including arthritis. The plant has shown some anti-inflammatory activity which may be attributed to its salicylic acid content. Potential problems with ulcer formation is reduced by its triterpene racemoside which has antiulcer activity. It also contains other triterpenes including cimigoside and actein. Actein increases peripheral circulation.

Dandelion (*Taraxacum officinale*) plant is identified with its cholagogue and diuretic activity. These excretory functions make it applicable for chronic rheumatic conditions also. The bitter triterpene alcohols amyrin, taraxerol, and taraxasterol are considered to be the components responsible for its activity. Amyrin has shown anti-inflammatory effects. Another compound found abundantly in the roots, leaves, and flowers is sitosterol. Sitosterol has anti-inflammatory and antifever actions similar to cortisone and aspirin, respectively. However, sitosterol has a wide margin of safety compared to these drugs.

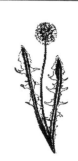

The need for controlling inflammation varies according to the severity of pain and loss of function. Severe, acute inflammation requires more frequent doses than milder chronic problems. The appropriate dosage range is therefore broad and the usual dose of 15-30 drops can be used from one to six times daily.

Add one of the following formulas if needed.

Alterative Formula

The underlying condition leading to much rheumatic pain has been addressed in the past by utilizing herbal means for enhancing elimination of metabolic waste. By improving the quality of the nourishing fluids that surround the cells and tissues of the musculoskeletal system, normal function is supported and irritating influences are reduced. Inflammation is relieved as irritation subsides.

Analgesic and Antispasmodic Formula

When the discomfort and dysfunction associated with connective tissue inflammation excessively limits normal activity, using herbs that specifically relieve pain and spasm can help tremendously. While activity should still be restrained in such conditions, the unnecessary suffering associated with regular or severe pain need not simply be tolerated. Even partial palliation of a constant ache can aid in relaxation and result in significant relief of the mental anguish often associated with intractable pain.

GETTING FIT AND STAYING ACTIVE

AID IN RECOVERING FROM ACUTE INJURIES AND CHRONIC INFLAMMATORY CONDITIONS

Physical Therapy	Cramps	Joint Sprains	Muscle Strains	Bruises	Bursitis	Tendinitis	Arthritis	Fibromyositis
Massage	•	♣	•	♣	♣			•
Manipulation	•		♣					•
Heat	•	♣	•	♣		•	•	•
Rest	•	•	•		•	•	•	•
Ice		✳	✳	✳	✳			
Electrical Stimulation	•							•
Diathermy		♣		♣	♣	•	•	•
Ultrasound		♣	•	♣	•	•	•	•

TOPICAL HERBAL OILS OR EXTRACTS

	Cramps	Joint Sprains	Muscle Strains	Bruises	Bursitis	Tendinitis	Arthritis	Fibromyositis
Camphor	•				•	•	•	•
Wintergreen	•				•	•	•	•
Peppermint	•				•	•	•	•
Eucalyptus	•				•	•	•	•
Cinnamon	•				•	•	•	•
Cayenne	•				•	•	•	•
Arnica		•	•	•				
Calendula		•	•	•				
Comfrey		•	•	•				
St.Johnswort		•	•	•				
Witch Hazel		•	•	•				

♣ Denotes a 'later' treatment only.

✳ Denotes an 'early' treatment only.

KEEPING THE MUSCULOSKELETAL SYSTEM IN TOP SHAPE

Muscular Strengthening	Avoiding Injuries	Relieving Painful Spasms	Reducing Inflammation
Physical Labor	Regular Activity	Black Cohosh	Devils Claw
Strenuous Exercise	Physical	Kava Kava	Yucca
Athletics	Examination	Jamaica Dogwood	Black Cohosh
Balanced Activities	Moderation	Ginger	Dandelion
	Keep Weight	Calcium	Ginger
	Down	Magnesium	Bromelain
	Proper	Contract Opposing	Papain
	Equipment	Muscle Group	
	Stretching/		
	Warming Up		
	Recognize		
	Limitations		
	Avoid Drug Use		

IX

SURFACE INFECTIONS

Skin And Alimentary Mucosa

The skin and mucosa coverings provide protection for the internal body from infections. They are assisted in this by lymphatic tissue which destroys invading microorganisms. Preserving the integrity of these tissues, practicing good hygiene, and promoting the growth of healthy bacteria helps insure against the establishment of disease microbes.

The skin is the largest organ of the body. It serves as an organ since it provides unique and necessary functions for the body. **The skin helps regulate the body temperature by the amount of blood flowing near the surface and by the evaporation of perspiration.** Hot, dry skin is associated with high fevers. Sweating not only helps to control fevers, but it aids in eliminating salts and keeping the skin healthy. **The skin also forms a barrier which limits fluid loss and the penetration into the body of external substances and microorganisms.** When breaks in the skin surface provide access to body tissues, white blood cells consume invading bacteria and prevent them from spreading through the body. **If microbes do penetrate deep into tissues they are filtered out of the lymph and destroyed in lymph nodes.** When they succeed in entering the blood they are usually consumed in the spleen and bone marrow.

In addition to requiring contact with a disease-producing microbial agent, infections of the skin are commonly due to poor immunity in an individual. "Opportunistic" infections occur in response to a general systemic condition which lowers overall resistance. Such predisposing factors as diabetes, kidney failure, leukemia, or drug therapies using cortisone or other immune suppressants increase the risk of infection. **The skin's ability to resist infection is also highly dependant upon local skin conditions.** Poor local blood circulation, particularly in the extremities, leads to the development of chronic infections and poor wound healing in the area. Wounds, burns, ulcers, or other open lesions of the skin increase the likelihood of bacterial infection. Local cleansing and antiseptic applications are beneficial in these cases. Yeast and fungus infections are more likely to occur in areas that remain damp or moist. These include the groin area, between the toes, in the ear canal, and under large breasts in women. Keeping moisture from remaining on the skin is important. This can be aided by wearing loose cotton clothing rather than synthetic. The moisture is better absorbed and can evaporate as the air circulates freely next to the skin. Exposure to sunlight or other sources of ultraviolet radiation is deadly for many microbes. However, since ultraviolet rays do not pass through material their effectiveness is blocked by clothing, hair, scabs, flaking skin, or other physical obstacles.

Like the skin covering the external surface of the body, the inner surface of the alimentary canal (the tract from the mouth to the anus) is lined with mucosa (a mucous membrane surface). The throat and its mucosa are also part of the respiratory tract.

The throat area is a common site for infections because of its exposure to dry air, irritating substances, and bacteria from outside. **The lymphoid tissue called Waldeyer's ring that circles the throat helps protect the middle ear, digestive tract, and lower respiratory tract from infections.** It consists of the tonsils, adenoids, and tonsilar tissues at the base of the tongue and around the auditory tubes. In children these lymphoid tissues may enlarge and block the internal opening to the auditory tube. This predisposes to middle ear infections. Enlargement of local lymph nodes can block drainage of the ears, nose, and throat area, aggravating local congestive symptoms. Chronic infections of this area often occur when allergies increase mucus production and congestion.

Ideally, all infections should be controlled early in their course to avoid complications. The common cold is caused by a virus, but frequently it leads to bacterial infections of the ears, nose, throat, or lungs. Bacteria can spread from throat infections to these other organs and vice versa. When sore throats are beginning it is helpful to use a heating compress at bedtime. This is done by wrapping a cold, wet cotton cloth around the neck. This compress is then completely covered with a thick, snug (not tight) wrapping of flannel or wool (such as a large wool sock) which is held in place with safety pins. The cold cloth activates a circulatory response which increases blood flow in the area. This produces local heat and reduces congestion. This heating compress is kept in place overnight or until it is dry. **Lymph drainage to reduce congestion in the throat can be enhanced by lymphatic massage techniques.** Externally, the flat of the hand is slowly drawn from just below the ear down the side of neck to the collar bone and held

there for a moment. This should be done repeatedly.
If lymph node swelling and congestion in the postna-
sal area block the internal opening of the auditory
tube, it can be opened by an oral internal massage
technique known as endonasal therapy. This clinical
procedure helps to prevent or resolve middle ear
infections.

In terms of its surface area the alimentary mucosa, equal to the size of two tennis courts, is even
larger than the skin. While this mucosa selectively
secretes enzymes and fluids and absorbs nutrients
and water, it also serves to separate waste and the
intestinal microbes from the rest of the body. **The
mucosal lining of the gut provides both a physical
and an immune barrier.** The normal intestinal bacterial count far outnumbers all of the cells that com-
pose the body. Viruses, yeast, or amebic parasites
might also be present. **Lymph tissue is found
throughout the intestinal mucosa in areas called
Peyer's patches and in the appendix at the opening
where the colon begins. These lymph tissues help to
block the entry of these microorganism into the
body.** Toxins and bacteria that do penetrate the
intestinal mucosa are carried by the portal blood to
the liver. Here special phagocytes destroy the bacteria. Microorganisms are thereby safely contained in
the intestinal tract and kept separate from the rest of
the body's tissues. Food allergies can impair immune
efficiency by weakening the protective barrier provided by the mucosa and the lymph tissue.

**The bowels usually suffer infections due to poor
hygienic practices.** The infections associated with the
gastrointestinal tract are often referred to as "intestinal flu" though they are usually caused by gram-
negative bacteria and not by viruses. Intestinal
inflammation is sometimes due to bacterial toxins in

spoiled food that affect the bowels. Poorly cooked poultry is a source of the bacteria that produce nausea, vomiting, bloating, cramps, diarrhea, and/or fever or headaches. Another common reason for intestinal infections is inadequate cleanliness of food handlers. This results in contamination of food with bacteria normally found in the colon. Dysentery with blood and mucus in the stools can be caused by either bacteria or protozoal parasites from contaminated food or water. Extreme diarrhea requires fluid and mineral replacement to avoid circulatory complications.

When intestinal bacteria are killed by antibiotic drugs an overgrowth of Candida yeast can become established in the alimentary mucosa. The prolonged use of birth control pills or cortisone and the excessive consumption of sugar have also been associated with this yeast infection. It can cause irritable bowels, indigestion, and gas. Candida infections have been suspected of contributing to food allergies and immune reactions. Associated conditions include migraines, rheumatoid arthritis, asthma, depression, PMS, and chronic fatigue. Control of this chronic infection involves avoidance in the diet of certain food or drinks including articles containing other yeasts (breads and natural vitamin B-complex), sugars (table sugar, corn syrup, molasses, and honey), and fermented substances (alcoholic beverages, aged cheese, soy sauce). **Consuming sources of live acidophilus cultures such as yogurt helps to re-establish the dominance of good bacteria in the gut.** Candida commonly causes oral, groin, and vaginal yeast infections, also. Cultured milk products with live acidophilus will compete with vaginal Candida overgrowth and produce lactic acid to acidify the vagina. Vaginal douching once or twice daily can be done with one of several dilute solutions (1 cup of buttermilk or unsweetened yogurt per quart of distilled water). Acidifying the vagina by daily douching with 3-5 tablespoons of distilled vinegar per quart of warm water can help to temporarily relieve the itching caused by local yeast or trichomonal protozoa infections. Retention douches with an iodine solution inhibits the growth of Candida and Trichomonas.

Antifungal and Antiyeast Formula

While most surface fungus infections occur on the skin or nails, the single-celled form of fungus known as yeast commonly infect mucous membranes as well as the skin. Infections that occur on the skin can usually be treated with simple local applications. If there is an open sore or the tissue is irritated or sensitive, it will be necessary to dilute an alcohol-based preparation with water to avoid aggravating the discomfort. For external conditions such as these, one part of an alcoholic extract mixed with four parts water should prevent further irritation. For infections confined to a small spot, a cotton ball moistened with the dilution can be held in place with a bandaid. The dilution should be applied frequently using cotton if the area involved is too large or constant contact cannot be maintained as in the case of fungal infections of the feet. For an infection of the nails the formula can be combined with distilled vinegar and used daily to soak the toes or fingertips.

Yerba mansa (*Anemopsis californica*) root is a Southwestern herb that was used topically to treat sores. The root contains an aromatic oil that contains mostly methyleugenol but also has significant amounts of thymol. Methyleugenol is moderately antimicrobial against certain yeast and fungus as well as some gram-positive and a few gram-negative bacteria. Thymol is very active at inhibiting these microorganisms.

Black walnut (*Juglans nigra*) green hulls have been used topically in cases of ringworm (fungus) and herpes (virus) and internally for worms. The fresh hulls contain high concentrations of the naphtho-quinone juglone and a number of similar derivatives. Though juglone inhibits some yeast, gram-positive bacteria, and acid-fast bacteria, it is most active against fungus. It has been shown to be very effective against fungal skin infections when it is used locally. Juglone also has shown limited antiviral activity.

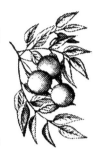

Pau d'arco (*Tabebuia spp.*) inner bark is an excellent remedy for infections and has recently become popular for controlling yeast overgrowth. It contains a variety of active naphthoquinones of which lapachol, xyloidone, lapachone, and dehydro-lapachone are prominent in the various species. As antibacterial agents, lapachol and lapachone inhibit the growth of certain gram-positive bacteria, while they and the others strongly inhibit the gram-nega-tive Brucella bacteria, also. Lapachol has some antiviral activity. Extracts of pau d'arco have shown a distinct anti-inflammatory effect as well.

Usnea (*Usnea barbata*) is a lichen that grows from trees. It contains the antibacterial compounds atranorin and usnic acid. Usnic acid has shown antimicrobial activity against certain fungus and gram-positive bacteria. It is also anti-inflammatory. Usnic acid is not absorbed well from the gut, so it can be useful for infections of the intestines.

This combination is active on contact against fungus, yeast, and bacteria, so it is especially useful for external infections. Since several of these herbs inhibit Candida, it can also be used orally in cases of yeast infections involving the mouth, intestines, or vagina. Most of the bacteria it inhibits are gram-positive which won't disrupt the largely gram-negative flora normally found in the intestines. As a mouthwash 15 - 30 drops can be mixed with a small amount of water and used from one to five times daily to control thrush, a yeast infection of the mouth. This solution can also be swallowed to inhibit the Candida that are likely to be flourishing in the intestines as well. Using the extract orally can aid in controlling local chronic or recurring Candida infections of the vagina or groin area by reducing the shedding of yeast from the bowels. **Alcoholic extracts should not be used in vaginal douches.**

Add the following formula if needed.

Antiseptic Formula

If one formula is not sufficiently effective to control a local infection, adding the other can improve the results. This combination is also appropriate internally for intestinal infections that involve yeast or bacteria. Each formula contains herbs whose activity is due to their unique constituents. These constituents have different activities and cover a broader range more effectively when combined. Combining the formulas is not always necessary but can be helpful in particular cases.

Antiseptic Formula

Inflammation of the mucous membrane surface of the throat and the intestines is often a result of microbial infections. The throat is a common site for viral and bacterial proliferation, while bacteria and protozoa are a common cause of acute diarrhea and dysentery. The overuse of antibiotics has led increasingly to bacteria that develop resistance to their effects. When broad-spectrum antibiotics are relied upon, it increases the danger of eliminating enough friendly bacteria to allow Candida yeast to flourish. To avoid the proliferation of yeast and prevent bacterial or parasitic infections from progressing, herbal antiseptics that inhibit bacteria, yeast, and protozoa can be employed for infections of the mucosa. Whereas antibiotics often interfere with the immune response while eliminating bacteria, herbal enhancement of the immune response can help the body to overcome infections of all types.

Goldenseal (*Hydrastis canadensis*) root has been used to treat inflamed mucous membranes where there is an excessive amount of mucus production. Its local antiseptic use has been applied to both skin and mucosal infections. Besides the major active alkaloids berberine and hydrastine, goldenseal contains a number of others including hydrastinine. Berberine, hydrastine, and hydrastinine each inhibit certain gram-negative bacteria. Berberine is the most potent of these. It has been found to also inhibit the growth of a number of gram-positive bacteria, yeast, fungus, and protozoa. Berberine also prevents certain pathologic gram-positive and gram-negative infectious bacteria from sticking to the mucosa. Berberine not only blocks diarrhea caused by bowel toxins from certain bacteria, but oral treatment for intestinal infections with Candida yeast and Giardia or Entamoeba protozoa was effective. Since much of the berberine is not absorbed from the gut, its use for intestinal problems is appropriate. Berberine has been found to be safe and effective in treating diarrhea in infants, children, and adults. It also has anti-inflammatory activity.

Narrow-leafed echinacea (*Echinacea angustifolia*) root has been used for skin and throat infections locally and internally, as well as being taken internally for respiratory and intestinal infections. Antibacterial activity has been shown for its echinacoside component. Polyacetylenes from the root inhibited various gram-positive and gram-negative bacteria, Candida yeast, and fungus. The greatest benefit of echinacea alcoholic extract, however, may be provided by the immune stimulant activity of isobutylamides, echinacoside, and cynarin from the root. High molecular weight polysaccharides from water extracts of the root have shown both immune-enhancing and anti-inflammatory effects. These polysaccharides are probably responsible for blocking the enzyme hyaluronidase which bacteria use to penetrate into tissues. A tea made from the root makes an excellent vehicle to dilute alcohol-based extracts for application to the skin.

For throat infections the extract should be diluted slightly for gargling and then swallowed. It can simply be mixed in a liquid vehicle and swallowed for problems caused by bacteria in the intestines. Normally, it should be used three times each day between meals. The time required to rid the intestines of disease microbes can be prolonged because the area involved is extensive. To eliminate protozoa the use of herbs should continue beyond the disappearance of symptoms. To avoid a relapse, lab tests can be done to examine the stool for the absence of parasites to indicate when the treatment has been completely successful. Topical application for infections requires dilution of the alcoholic extract with water to avoid irritation. **(Alcoholic extracts should never be used in the eye nor in a douche for nasal, sinus, or vaginal membranes.)** Internal administration of the extract should accompany its external use.

Add one of the following formulas if needed.

Carminative Antacid and Flavoring Formula

When used internally, the goldenseal extract has a strong bitter taste that many find unpleasant. Using the flavoring formula as a vehicle to "carry" the antiseptics makes the medicating experience much more tolerable. Together with the sweetness of the glycerin, the peppermint and cinnamon flavors go a long way in helping to mask the bitterness.

Antifungal and Antiyeast Formula

Since certain herbs are sometimes limited in their ability to inhibit the growth of particular microbes, using a number of herbs together can be more effective in limiting the offending germs. Both the antiseptic and antifungal herbal combinations affect a variety of both bacteria and fungus. When used together they have a more potent impact in controlling the growth of infectious agents.

Ear Canal Formula

Infections of the middle ear can be addressed with dietary, antibacterial, and immune therapies. To prevent the build-up of pressure and possible rupture, it also helps to keep the internal auditory tube open to allow drainage. Reducing the congestion in Waldeyer's ring in the throat by inhibiting the bacteria there helps to assure the drainage is maintained. Gargling with this antiseptic solution also protects the throat so that infection does not spread back and forth. After gargling this antiseptic formula should be swallowed to help improve immune function.

Ear Canal Formula

Wax production in the ear canal is usually not a problem; however, sometimes the wax hardens and cannot be expelled. When wax build-up is excessive, water can become trapped in the ear canal. If showering or swimming results in moisture retention as a regular occurrence, the ear canal provides an opportune location for fungus to grow (the so-called "swimmer's ear). This local infection can produce itching or pain and result in further adherence of the wax to the walls of the canal. To soften the wax so that it can be released, an oil-based antifungal preparation is ideal for local use. The oil can better penetrate into the surface and ease pain when it is warmed first. Herbal antiseptics extracted in the oil can also inhibit bacterial and viral growth. The use of antiseptic oil to prevent microbial growth in the ear canal may also be of benefit early in the course of middle ear infections. These antiseptic ear drops are not intended for oral use. They are for external use only. Ear drops should never be used in the ear canal if there is a discharge coming from a ruptured ear drum. A doctor's exam is necessary if this occurs.

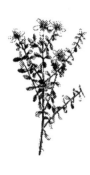

St. Johnswort (*Hypericum perforatum*) flowers are prepared for local use by extracting them while still fresh with olive oil. The flowers cause the oil to turn a deep red. This oil has been used externally as a vulnerary for burns, wounds, sores, and other skin problems and to relieve pain. The flowers are rich in flavonoids that have demonstrated pain-relieving and antimicrobial activity. St. Johnswort flowers also contain a bicyclic tetraketone called hyperforin which effectively inhibits topical infections caused by common gram-positive bacteria. The flower's polycyclic dione components hypericin and pseudohypericin have shown potent antiviral activity against retroviruses.

Mullein (*Verbascum thapsus*) flowers have been used internally as a demulcent and externally to relieve inflammation and painful skin conditions.

The mucilage from the flowers is made up of polysaccharides soluble in the extract's glycerine base. The
oil extracted from the flowers has been used in the ear
canal for loss of hearing due to the secretion of wax.
This oil applied to the ear drum is believed to have a
relaxing effect. The flowers also contain derivatives
of flavonoid glycosides having anti-inflammatory
effects. Another of its flavonoids, 3'-
methylquercetin, has shown antiviral activity. Mullein flowers extracts inhibit the growth of influenza
viruses by stimulating interferon-like activity.

Garlic (*Allium sativa*) bulbs (cloves) have commonly been used for internal infections. Garlic
extracts inhibit a wide variety of infectious agents.
After being crushed the bulbs release a volatile
component, allicin, which inhibits common skin
fungi and Candida yeast. Higher levels of allicin are
needed to kill certain gram-positive and gram-
negative bacteria. Crushed garlic also contains other
antimicrobial thiosulphinate components, and anti-
Candida ajoenes are found in the oil extract. Garlic
juice mixed with oil and glycerin has been used in the
ear for hearing difficulties due to excessive wax or
chronic problems of the mucous tissues in the ear.

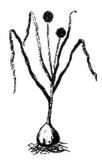

The solvents for this formula are glycerin and
olive oil. No alcohol is present that would cause
irritation to inflamed surfaces in the ear canal. This
remedy is used 5-10 drops at a time in the external ear
canal from one to three times daily. The oil may be
warmed by holding a glass dropper filled with the oil
under hot running water from the tap for five to ten
seconds. The end of the dropper will need to be held
shut to avoid letting the warm oil run out the opening
in the tip. Another method of warming the oil is to
heat a clean metal spoon in hot tap water and then
put the drops in the spoon for a few seconds before

placing them in the ear canal. Once the drops are put in the ear canal a cotton plug is inserted to prevent the oil from draining out. The ear being treated should be kept facing upwards as long as possible to retain the antiseptic oil. Bedtime is usually the most convenient time to do this. For ear pain associated with fever and sinus congestion or a sore throat, the internal use of other remedies may also be necessary. Add the following formula if needed.

Antiseptic Formula

When there is a topical infection in the ear canal, the application locally of antibacterial and antifungal herbs helps to eradicate the problematic microorganism. While the ear oil can inhibit the growth of certain microbes, its effectiveness when used together with other antiseptics is greater and wider. The antiseptics can also be used in water as a gargle to address associated throat conditions.

REDUCING SUPERFICIAL MICROBIAL GROWTH

CAUSES AND CONTROL OF MICROBIAL PROLIFERATION

Susceptible Skin	Skin Support	Vulnerable Membranes	Membrane Support
Burns	Cotton Clothing	Dryness	Heating
Wounds	Sunshine	Irritants	Compress
Ulcers	Cleansing	Lymph Conges-	Lymphatic
Penetration by	Local Antisepsis	tion	Massage
Microbes		Contamination	Dietary Care
Diabetes		of Air/ Food/	Cultured Milk
Kidney Failure		Water	(Oral or Vaginal)
Leukemia		Allergies	Vaginal Douching:
Steroid Use		Antibiotics	Diluted Vinegar
Poor Circulation		Birth Control	Iodine Solution
Chronic Moistness		Pills	
		Steroids	
		Excessive Sugars	

ANTIMICROBIAL HERB APPLICATIONS

Fungus/Yeast/ Bacteria	Bacteria/Protozoa/ Yeast/Fungus	Fungus/Yeast/ Bacteria/Virus
Topical	Internal	External
(and/or internal)	(and/or topical)	(ear canal only)
Yerba Mansa	Goldenseal	St.Johnswort
Black Walnut	Echinacea	Mullein
Pau d'Arco		Garlic
Usnea		

REFERENCES

Books:

All Chapters

Alstat E (ed.), *Eclectic Dispensatory of Botanical Therapeutics,* vol. 1, Eclectic Medical Publications, Portland, Oregon, 1989

Felter HW & Lloyd JU, *King's American Dispensatory,* 18th ed., 3rd rev., Eclectic Medical Publications, Portland, Oregon, 1983

Lust J, *The Herb Book,* Bantam Books, Inc., New York, New York, 1974

Priest AW & Priest LR, *Herbal Medication,* L.N. Fowler & Co. Ltd., London, England, 1982

Weiss RF, *Herbal Medicine,* Beaconsfield Publishers Ltd., Beaconsfield, England, 1988

Journals:

I CLEANSING & IMMUNITY

Alterative Formula

Anonymous - Limonene trial in cancer, *Lancet,* 342:801, 1993

Abe N et al., Interferon Induction by Glycyrrhizin and Glycyrrhetinic Acid in Mice, *Microbiol. Immunol.,* 26:535-539, 1982

Adolf W. & Hecker E, New Irritant Diterpene-Esters from Roots of Stillingia Sylvatica L. (Euphorbiaceae), *Tetrahedron Lett.,* 21:2887-90, 1980

Amin AH et al., Berberine sulfate : antimicrobial activity, bioassay, and mode of action, *Can. J. Microbiol.,* 15:1067-76, 1969

Anderson DM & Smith WG, The Antitussive Activity of Glycyrrhetinic Acid and its Derivatives, *J. Pharm. Pharmacol.,* 13:396-404, 1961

Belkin M et al., Swelling and Vacuolization Induced in Ascites Tumor Cells by Polysaccharides from Higher Plants, *Cancer Res.,* 19:1050-62, 1959

Boyd EM, Expectorants and Respiratory Tract Fluid, *Pharmacol. Rev.,* 6:521-42, 1954

Chan MY, The Effect of Berberine on Bilirubin Excretion in the Rat, *Comp. Med. East West,* 5:161-8, 1977

Crombie L, Amides of Vegetable Origin. Part III. Structure and Stereo chemistry of neoHerculin, *J. Chem. Soc.,* pp. 995-8, 1955

Fairbairn JW, Anthracene derivatives of natural occurrence, *Pharmaceut. J.,* pp. 271-4, March 30, 1963

Fish F & Waterman PG, Alkaloids in the bark of Zanthoxylum clava-
herculis, *J. Pharm. Pharmac.*, 25:115P-6P, 1973

Foldeak S & Dombradi GA, Tumor-growth inhibiting substances of plant
origin. I. Isolation of the active principle of Arctium lappa, *Acta Univ.
Szeged., Acta Phys. Chem.*, 10:91-3, 1964

Gupte S, Use of Berberine in Treatment of Giardiasis, *Am. J. Dis. Child.*,
129:866, 1975

Hoerhammer L et al., New methods in pharmacognostical education. XIII.
Thin-layer chromatography of components of Rhamnus cortical
drugs and their preparation, *Deut. Apoth.-Ztg.*, 107:563-6, 1967
(*Chem. Abs.* 67:84920u)

Hulme A & Bateson MC, Complications of Carbenoxolone Therapy, *Br.
Med. J.*, p. 804, Sep. 28, 1974

Kazakov AL et al., Flavonoids of the genus Trifolium, *Khim. Prir. Soedin.*,
9:432-3, 1973 (*Chem. Abs.* 79:102793j)

Kitagawa K et al., Inhibition of the Specific Binding of 12-O-
Tetradecanoylphorbol-13-Acetate to Mouse Epidermal Membrane
Fractions by Glycyrrhetic Acid, *Oncology*, 43:127-30, 1986

Kumazawa Y et al., Activation of Peritoneal Macrophages by Berberine-
type Alkaloids in Terms of Induction of Cytostatic Activity, *Int. J.
Immunopharmac.*, 6:587-92, 1984

Lenfeld J et al., Antiinflammatory Activity of Quaternary
Benzophenanthridine Alkaloids from Chelidonium majus, *Planta
Med.*, 43:161-5, 1981

McKenna GF & Taylor A, Screening Plant Extracts for Anticancer
Activity, *Tex. Rep. Biol. Med.*, 20:214-20, 1962

Mitscher LA et al., Antimicrobial Agents from Higher Plants. I. Introduc
tion, Rationale, and Methodology, *Lloydia*, 35:157-66, 1972

Mitscher LA et al., Antimicrobial Agents from Higher Plants. Antimicro
bial Isoflavanoids and Related Substances from Glycyrrhiza Glabra L.
Var. Typica, *J. Nat. Prod.*, 43:259-69, 1980

Morita K et al., A desmutagenic factor isolated from burdock (Arctium
lappa Linne), *Mutat. Res.*, 129:25-31, 1984

Murdock KE & Allen WE, Germicidal Effect of Orange Peel Oil and D-
Limonene in Water and Orange Juice, *Food Technol.*, 14:441-5, 1960

Nishino H et al., Antitumor-promoting activity of glycyrrhetic acid in
mouse skin tumor formation induced by 7,12-
dimethylbenz[a]anthracene plus teleocidin, *Carcinogen.*, 5:1529-30,
1984

Otsuka H et al., Studies on anti-inflammatory agents. II. Anti-inflamma
tory constituents from rhizome of Coptis japonica Makine, *Yaku.
Zasshi*, 101:883-90, 1981 (*Chem. Abs.* 96:28395p)

Pompei R et al., Glycyrrhizic acid inhibits virus growth and inactivates
virus particles, *Nature*, 281:690, 1979

Pompei R et al., Antiviral activity of glycyrrhizic acid, *Experientia,* 36:304, 1980

Rabbani GH et al., Randomized Controlled Trial of Berberine Sulfate Therapy for Diarrhea Due to Enterotoxigenic Escherichia coli and Vibrio cholerae, *J. Infect. Dis.,* 155:979-84, 1987

Reisch J et al., The Problem of the Microbiological Activity of Simple Acetylene Compounds, *Arzneim.-Forsch.,* 17:816-25, 1967

Russin WA et al., Inhibition of rat mammary carcinogenesis by monoterpenoids, *Carcinogen. (Lond.),* 10:2161-4, 1989

Steele VE et al., Inhibition of transformation in cultured rat tracheal epithelial cells by potential chemopreventive agents, *Canc. Res.,* 50:2068-74, 1990

Subba MS et al., Antimicrobial Action of Citrus Oils, *J. Food Sci.,* 32:225-7, 1967

Subbaiah TV & Amin AH, Effect of Berberine Sulphate on Entamoeba histolytica, *Nature,* 215, 527-8, 1967

Suess TR & Stermitz FR, Alkaloids of Mahonia Repens with a Brief Review of Previous Work in the Genus Mahonia, *J. Nat. Prod.,* 44:680-7, 1981

Takeda S et al., Kidney disorder-treating agents containing guaiaretic acid, meso-dihydroguaiaretic acid, arctiin, arctigenine, or asarinin, *Chem. Abs.,*113:410, 1990 (#103446f)

Tangri KK et al., Biochemical Study of Anti-inflammatory and Anti-arthritic Properties of Glycyrrhetic Acid, *Biochem Pharmacol.,* 14:1277-81, 1965

Taylor A et al., Anticancer Activity of Plant Extracts, *Tex. Rep. Biol. Med.,* 14:538-56, 1956

Terracciano M et al., HPLC analytical study of the principal constituents of cascara and frangula extracts, *Boll. Chim. Farm.,* 116:402-9, 1977 (*Chem. Abs.* 88:110563k)

Turova AD et al., Berberine, an effective cholagogue, *Med. Prom. SSSR,* 18:59-60, 1964 (*Chem. Abs.* 61:15242f)

Velluda CC et al., Effect of Berberis vulgaris extract, and of the berberine, berbamine, and oxyacanthine alkaloids on liver and bile function, *Lucra. prez. conf. natl. farm.,* Bucharest, pp. 351-4, 1958 (*Chem. Abs.* 53:15345a)

Wash LK & Bernard JD, Licorice-induced Pseudoaldosteronism, *Am. J. Hosp. Pharm.,* 32:73-4, 1975

Zukerman I, Effect of Oxidized d-Limonene on Micro-organisms, *Nature,* 168:517, 1951

Immune Support Formula

Bauer R et al., Immunological in vivo and in vitro Examinations of

Echinacea Extracts, *Arzneim.-Forsch.,* 38:276-81, 1988

Bauer R et al., TLC and HPLC Analysis of Echinacea pallida and E. angustifolia Roots, *Planta Med.,* 54:426-30, 1988

Bauer R et al., Alkamides from the Roots of Echinacea purpurea, *Phytochem.,* 27:2339-42, 1988

Bauer R & Remiger P, TLC and HPLC Analysis of Alkamides in Echinacea Drugs, *Planta Med.,* 55:367-71, 1989

Bauer R et al., Alkamides and Caffeic Acid Derivatives from the Roots of Echinacea tennesseensis, *Planta Med.,* 56:533-4, 1990

Bohlmann F & Hoffmann H, Further amides from Echinacea purpurea, *Phytochem.,* 22:1173-5, 1983

Cheminat A et al., Caffeoyl Conjugates from Echinacea Species: Structures and Biological Activity, *Phytochem.,* 27:2787-94, 1988

Heinzer F et al., Classification of the therapeutically used species of the genus Echinacea, *Pharm. Acta Helv.,* 63:132-6, 1988 (*Chem. Abs.* 109:146331z)

Kiso Y et al., Assay Method for Antihepatotoxic Activity Using Macrophage-mediated Cytotoxicity in Primary Cultured Hepatocytes, *Phytother. Res.,* 1:61-4, 1987

Luettig B et al., Macrophage activation by the polysaccharide arabinogalactan isolated from plant cell cultures of Echinacea purpurea, *J. Natl. Cancer Inst.,* 81:669-75, 1989

May G & Willuhn G, Antiviral Activity of Aqueous Extracts from Medicinal Plants in Tissue Cultures, *Arzneim.-Forsch.,* 28:1-7, 1978

Meibner FK, Experimental Studies of the Mode of Action of a Herba recens Echinaceae purpureae on Skin Flap, *Arzneim.-Forsch.,* 37:17-20, 1987

Orinda D et al., Antiviral Activity of Compounds of Echinacea purpurea, *Arzneim.-Forsch.,* 23:1119-20, 1973

Roesler J et al., Application of purified polysaccharides from cell cultures of the plant Echinacea purpurea to mice mediates protection against systemic infections with Listeria monocytogenes and Candida albicans, *Int. J. Immunopharmacol.,* 13:27-37, 1991

Schulte KE et al., The Presence of Polyacetylene Compounds in Echinacea purpurea Mnch. and Echinacea angustifolia DC, *Arzneim.-Forsch.,* 17:825-9, 1967

Tubaro A et al., Anti-inflammatory activity of a polysaccharidic fraction of Echinacea angustifolia, *J. Pharm. Pharmacol.,* 39:567-9, 1987

Tunnerhoff FK & Schwabe HK, Studies in Human Beings and Animals on the Influence of Echinacea Extracts on the Formation of Connective Tissue following the Implantation of Fibrin, *Arzneim.-Forsch.,* 6:330-4, 1956

Voaden DJ & Jacobson M, Tumor Inhibitors. 3. Identification and
    Synthesis of an Oncolytic Hydrocarbon from American Coneflower
    Roots, *J. Med. Chem.*, 15:619-23, 1972
Vogel G et al., The Problem of the Evaluation of Antiexsudative Drugs,
    Arzneim.-Forsch., 18:426-9, 1968
Vomel T, Influence of a Vegetable Immune Stimulant on Phagocytosis of
    Erythrocytes by the Reticulohistiocytary System of Isolated Perfused
    Rat Liver, *Arzneim.-Forsch.*, 35:1437-1440, 1985
Wacker A & Hilbig W, Virus inhibition by Echinacea purpurea, *Planta
    Med.*, 33:89-102, 1978
Wagner H et al., Immunostimulating Polysaccharides (Heteroglycans) of
    Higher Plants, *Arzneim.-Forsch.*, 35:1069-75, 1985
Zoutewelle G & van Wijk R, Effects of Echinacea purpurea Extracts on
    Fibroblast Populated Collagen Lattice Contraction, *Phytother. Res.*,
    4:77-81, 1990

II NUTRITION & DIGESTION

Bitter Digestive Tonic Formula

Amin AH et al., Berberine sulfate: antimicrobial activity, bioassay, and
    mode of action, *Can. J. Microbiol.*, 15:1067-76, 1969
Berezhinskaya VY et al., Anticholinesterase activity of some isoquinoline
    alkaloids, *Farmakol. Toksikol.*, 31:296-9, 1968 (*Chem. Abs.*
    69:50676v)
Bohm K, Studies on the Choleretic Action of some Drugs, *Arzneim.-
    Forsch.*, 9:376-8, 1959
Brogden RN et al., Deglycyrrhizinised Liquorice: A Report of Its Pharma
    cological Properties and Therapeutic Efficacy in Peptic Ulcer, *Drugs,*
    8:330-9, 1974
Doll R et al., Clinical Trial of a Triterpenoid Liquorice Compound in
    Gastric and Duodenal Ulcer, *Lancet*, pp. 793-6, Oct. 20, 1962
Forster HB et al., Antispasmodic Effects of Some Medicinal Plants, *Planta
    Med.*, 40:309-19, 1980
Garb S & Cattell M, A Study of the Effects of Bitters on the Growth of
    Rats, *Drug Stand.*, 24:94-8, 1956
Genest K & Hughes DW, Natural Products in Canadian Pharmaceuticals
    IV. Hydrastis Canadensis, *Can. J. Pharm. Sci.*, 4:41-5, 1969
Goetzl FR, Bitter Tonics I. Influence Upon Olfactory Acuity and Appe
    tite, *Drug Stand.*, 24:101-10, 1956
Goetzl FR, Bitter Tonics II. The Influence of Gentian Tincture Upon
    Gastric Evacuation, *Drug Stand.*, 24:111-4, 1956

Haranath PSRK et al., Acetylcholine and choline in common spices,
Phytother. Res., 1:91-2, 1987

Harkar S et al., Steroids, Chromone and Coumarins from Angelica
Officinalis, *Phytochem.,* 23:419-26, 1984

Harmala P et al., Isolation and Testing of the Calcium Blocking Activity of
Furanocoumarins from Angelica archangelica, *Planta Med.,* 57 (Suppl.
2):A58, 1991

Hayashi T & Kubo M, Anti-inflammatory secoiridoids, *Chem. Abs.,*
91:278, 1979 (#9485y)

Hulme A & Bateson MC, Complications of Carbenoxolone Therapy, *Br.
Med. J.,* p. 804, Sep. 28, 1974

Kassir ZA, Endoscopic controlled trial of four drug regimens in the
treatment of chronic duodenal ulceration, *Irish Med. J.,* 78:153-6, 1985

Kis I et al., Volatile terpenes from the roots of Angelica archangelica, *Rev.
Med. (Tirgu-Mures, Rom.),* 26:79-82, 1980 (*Chem. Abs.* 94:117799z)

Lewis JR, Carbenoxolone Sodium in the Treatment of Peptic Ulcer,
J.A.M.A., 229:460-2, 1974

Mansurov MM et al., Experimental effects of helenin on bleeding time and
the extent of blood loss, *Med. Zh. Uzb.,* (8):64-6, 1983 (*Chem. Abs.*
99:205851u)

Matsui M & Asai M, Analysis of menthone, isomenthone, anethole, and
cinnamaldehyde in crude drugs by headspace gas chromatography,
Shima. Hyo., 44:219-23, 1987 (*Chem. Abs.* 108:119050e)

Mori T et al., Effects of oral administration of glycyrrhizin and its
combinations on urine volume and electrolyte metabolism in rats,
Oyo Yakuri, 34:293-301, 1987 (*Chem. Abs.* 108:49307t)

Moersdorf K, Cyclic terpenes and their choleretic action, *Chim. Ther.,*
(7):442-3, 1966 (*Chem. Abs.* 66:74701p)

Niculesco G & Popesco M, The pharmacodynamic action of berberine,
Bull. Acad. Med. Roumanie, 17:210-5, 1945 (*Chem. Abs.* 41:5215i)

Niiho Y et al., Effects of a combined stomachic and its ingredients on
rabbit stomach motility in situ, *Jpn. J. Pharmacol.,* 27:177-9, 1977

Parke DV et al., The effects of ulcerogenic and ulcer-healing drugs on
gastric mucus, *Gut,* 16:396, 1975

Shinbo Y et al., Pharmaceuticals containing plant secoiridoids for treat
ment of gastritis and ulcer, *Chem. Abs.,* 111:318, 1989 (#28535n)

Takino Y et al., Quantitative Determination of Bitter Components in
Gentianaceous Plants, *Planta Med.,* 38:344-50, 1980

Tamas M & Popescu H, Determination of volatile components of Inulae
radix, fluid extract, *Farmacia (Bucharest),* 30:169-72, 1982 (*Chem.
Abs.* 98:77992f)

Turova AD et al., Berberine, *Lekarslv. Sredstva iz Rast.,* pp. 303-7, 1962
(*Chem Abs.* 58:2763b)

Turova AD et al., Berberine, an effective cholagogue, *Med. Prom. SSSR,*
18:59-60, 1964 (*Chem. Abs.* 61:15242f)

Velluda CC et al., Effect of Berberis vulgaris extract, and of the berberine,
berbamine, and oxyacanthine alkaloids on liver and bile function,
Sucr. prez. conf. natl. farm., Bucharest, pp. 351-4, 1958 (*Chem. Abs.*
53:15345a)

Wolf S & Mack M, Experimental Study of the Action of Bitters on the
Stomach of a Fistulous Human Subject, *Drug Stand.,* 24:98-101, 1956

Carminative Antacid and Flavoring Formula

Amin AH et al., Berberine sulfate: antimicrobial activity, bioassay, and
mode of action, *Can. J. Microbiol.,* 15:1067-1076, 1969

Evans BK et al., Further Studies on the Correlation Between Biological
Activity and Solubility of Some Carminatives, *J. Pharm. Pharmacol.,*
27(suppl.):66, 1975

Forster HB et al., Antispasmodic Effects of Some Medicinal Plants, *Planta
Med.,* 40:309-19, 1980

Gupte S, Use of Berberine in Treatment of Giardiasis, *Am. J. Dis. Child.,*
129:866, 1975

Kato T et al., Effects of a stomachic mixture on gastric secretion and
experimental ulcerations in rats, *Oyo Yak.,* 28:901-8, 1984 (*Chem.
Abs.* 102:55930h)

Kellner W & Kober W, The Possibility of using Ethereal Oils for the
Disinfection of Rooms, *Arzneim.-Forsch.,* 5:224-9, 1955

Maruzzella JC & Lichtenstein MB, The in Vitro Antibacterial Activity of
Oils, *J. Am. Pharm. Assoc.,* 45:378-81, 1956

Matsui M & Asai M, Analysis of menthone, isomenthone, anethole, and
cinnamaldehyde in crude drugs by headspace gas chromatography,
Shim. Hyoron, 44:219-23, 1987 (*Chem. Abs.* 108:119050e)

Moersdorf K, Cyclic terpenes and their choleretic action, *Chim. Ther.,*
(7):442-3, 1966 (*Chem. Abs.* 66:74701p)

Niiho Y et al., Effects of a Combined Stomachic and its Ingredients on
Rabbit Stomach Motility in Situ, *Japan. J. Pharmacol.,* 27:177-9, 1977

Nohara T et al., Constituents of Cinnamomi Cortex V. Structures of Five
Novel Diterpenes, Cinncassiols D_1, D_1 Glucoside, D_2, D_2 Glucoside
and D_3, *Chem. Pharm. Bull.,* 29:2451-9, 1981

Nohara T et al., Two Novel Diterpenes from Bark of Cinnamomum cassia,
Phytochem., 21:2130-2, 1982

Ohshima Y et al., High-performance liquid chromatographic separation of
rhubarb constituents, *J. Chromatogr.,* 360:303-6, 1986 (*Chem Abs.*
105:85251s)

Okuda T et al., Tannins of Medicinal Plants and Drugs, *Heterocycles,*
15:1323-48, 1981

Okuda T et al., Studies on the Activities of Tannins and Related Com
pounds from Medicinal Plants and Drugs. I. Inhibitory Effects on
Lipid Peroxidation in Mitochondria and Microsomes of Liver, *Chem.
Pharm. Bull.,* 31:1625-31, 1983

Oshio H & Noriaki K, Determination of the laxative components in
rhubarb by high performance liquid chromatography, *Shoyak. Zasshi,*
39:131-8, 1985 (*Chem. Abs.* 104:56493w)

Rabbani GH et al., Randomized controlled trial of berberine sulfate
therapy for diarrhea due to enterotoxigenic Escherichia coli and
Vibrio cholerae, *J. Infect. Dis.,* 155:979-84, 1987

Sharda KC, Berberine in the Treatment of Diarrhoea of Infancy and
Childhood, *J. Indian Med. Assoc.,* 54:22-4, 1970

Sigmund CJ & McNally EF, The Action of a Carminative on the Lower
Esophageal Sphincter, *Gastroenterol.,* 56:13-8, 1969

Subbaiah TV & Amin AH, Effect of Berberine Sulphate on Entamoeba
histolytica, *Nature,* 215:527-8, 1967

Tai Y-H et al., Antisecretory effects of berberine in rat ileum, *Am. J.
Physiol.,* 241:G253-8, 1981

Taylor BA et al., Inhibitory effect of peppermint oil on gastrointestinal
smooth muscle, *Gut,* 24:992, 1983

Turova AD et al., Berberine, *Lekarslv. Sredstva iz Rast.,* pp. 303-7, 1962
(*Chem. Abs.* 58:2763b)

Turova AD et al., Berberine, an effective cholagogue, *Med. Prom. SSSR,*
18:59-60, 1964 (*Chem. Abs.* 61:15242f)

Xiao P-G et al., Preliminary study on the correlation between phylogeny,
chemical constituents and therapeutic effects of Rheum species, *Yao
Hsueh Hsueh Pao,* 15:33-9, 1980 (*Chem. Abs.* 93:245330f)

Yagi A et al., The Constituents of Cinnamomi Cortex. I. Structures of
Cinncassiol A and Its Glucoside, *Chem. Pharm. Bull.,* 28:1432-6, 1980

III PROTECTION & ELIMINATION

Liver Tonic Formula

Besora C, Taraxacum Officinale, Weber, *Circ. Farm.,* 32:641-3, 1974

Bishop JG & Richardson AW, The Diphasic Actions of Ceanothyn and
EDTA as Blood Coagulants, *J. Am. Pharm. Assoc.,* 46:337-9, 1957

Bishop JG & Richardson AW, The Effect of Ceanothyn on Blood Coagu
lation Time, *J. Am. Pharm. Assoc.,* 46:396-8, 1957

Bohm K, Studies on the Choleretic Action of some Drugs, *Arzneim.-
Forsch.,* 9:376-8, 1959

Campos R et al., Silybin Dihemisuccinate Protects Against Glutathione
Depletion and Lipid Peroxidation Induced by Acetaminophen on Rat

Liver, *Planta Med.*, 55:417-9, 1989

Desplaces A et al., The Effects of Silymarin on Experimental Phalloidine Poisoning, *Arzneim.-Forsch.*, 25:89-96, 1975

Ferenci P et al., Randomized controlled trial of silymarin treatment in patients with cirrhosis of the liver, *J. Hepatol.*, 9:105-13, 1989

Gendrault JL et al., Behaviour of Liver Sinusoidal Cells Obtained from Silymarin-Treated Mice and Rats after in vivo and in vitro Infection with Frog Virus 3, *Planta Med.*, 39:247, 1980

Gupta MB et al., Anti-Inflammatory and Antipyretic Activities of b-Sitosterol, *Planta Med.*, 39:157-63, 1980

Hahn G et al., Pharmacology and Toxicology of Silymarin, the Antihepatotoxic Agent of Silybum marianum (L.) Gaertn., *Arzneim.-Forsch.*, 18:698-703, 1968

Hikino H et al., Antihepatotoxic Actions of Flavonolignans from Silybum marianum Fruits, *Planta Med.*, 50:248-50, 1984

Janiak B, Depression of microsomal activity in the liver of mice following single administration of halothane and its response to silybin, *Anaesthesist*, 23:389-93, 1974 (*Chem. Abs.* 82:11266k)

Lynch TA et al., An Investigation of the Blood Coagulating Principles from Ceanothus Americanus, *J. Am. Pharm. Assoc.*, 47:816-9, 1958

Magliulo E et al., Studies on the REgenerative Capacity of the Liver in Rats Subjected to Partial Hepatectomy and Treated with Silymarin, *Arzneim.-Forsch.*, 23:161-7, 1973

Mourelle M & Favari L, Silymarin Improves Metabolism and Dispostition of Aspirin in Cirrhotic Rats, *Life Sci.*, 43:201-7, 1988

Mourelle M et al., Protection Against Thallium Hepatotoxicity by Silymarin, *J. Appl. Toxicol.*, 8:351-4, 1988

Otsuka H et al., Studies on anti-inflammatory agents. II. Anti-inflammatory constituents from rhizome of Coptis japonica Makino, *Yaku. Zasshi*, 101:883-90, 1981 (*Chem. Abs.* 96:28395p)

Platt D & Schnorr B, Biochemical and Electronoptic Studies on the Possible Influence of Silymarin on Hepatic Damage Induced by Ethanol in Rats, *Arzneim.-Forsch.*, 21:1206-8, 1971

Racz-Kotilla E et al., The Action of Taraxacum Officinale Extracts on the Body Weight and Diuresis of Laboratory Animals, *Planta Med.*, 26:212-7, 1974

Salmi HA & Sarna S, Effect of silymarin on chemical, functional, and morphological alterations of the liver. A double-blind controlled study., *Scand. J. Gastroenterol.*, 17:417-21, 1982

Sarre H & Poser G, Experience in the Treatment of Chronic Hepatopathies with Silymarin, *Arzneim.-Forsch.*, 21:1209, 1971

Scheiber V & Wohlzogen FX, Analysis of a certain type of 2 X 3 tables, exemplified by biopsy findings in a controlled clinical trial, *Int. J. Clin. Pharmacol.*, 16:533-5, 1978

Servis RE et al., Peptide Alkaloids from Ceanothus americanus L. (Rhamnaceae), *J. Am. Chem. Soc.*, 91:5619-24, 1969

Suess TR & Stermitz FR, Alkaloids of Mahonia repens with a Brief Review of Previous Work in the Genus Mahonia, *J. Nat. Prod.*, 44:680-7, 1981

Susnik F, The Present State of Knowledge about the Medicinal Plant Taraxacum Officinale, *Med. Razgledi*, 21:323-8, 1982

Turova AD et al., Berberine, *Lekarslv. Sredstva iz Rast.*, pp. 303-7, 1962 (*Chem. Abs.* 58:2763b)

Turova AD et al., Berberine, an effective cholagogue, *Med. Prom. SSSR*, 18:59-60, 1964 (*Chem. Abs.* 61:15242f)

Valenzuela A et al., Silymarin protection against hepatic lipid peroxidation induced by acute ethanol intoxication in the rat, *Biochem. Pharm.*, 34:2209, 1985

Velluda CC et al., Effect of Berberis vulgaris extract, and of the berberine, berbamine, and oxyacanthine alkaloids on liver and bile function, *Lucra. prez. conf. natl. farm.*, *Bucharest*, pp. 351-4, 1958 (*Chem. Abs.* 53:15345a)

Virtanen P et al., Natural protoberberine alkaloids from Enantia chlorantha, palmatine, columbamine and jatrorrhizine for thioacetamide-traumatized rat liver, *Acta Anat.*, 131:166-70, 1988 (*Chem. Abs.* 108:198380p)

Vogel G et al., Protection by Silibinin against Amanita phalloides Intoxication in Beagles, *Toxicol. Appl. Pharmacol.*, 73:355-62, 1984

Wagner H et al., On Chemistry and Analysis of Silymarin from Silybum marianum Gaertn., *Arzneim.-Forsch.*, 24:466-71, 1974

Westerman L & Roddick JG, Annual Variation in Sterol Levels in Leaves of Taraxacum officinale Weber, *Plant Physiol.*, 68:872-5, 1981

Wolf S & Mack M, Experimental Study of the Action of Bitters on the Stomach of a Fistulous Human Subject, *Drug Stand.*, 24:98-101, 1956

Anthelmintic Formula

Albert-Puleo M, Mythobotany, Pharmacology, and Chemistry of Thujone-Containing Plants and Derivatives, *Econ. Bot.*, 32:65-74, 1978

Auyong TK et al., Pharmacological Aspects of Juglone, *Toxicon.*, 1:235-9, 1963

Clark, AM et al., Antimicrobial Activity of Juglone, *Phytother. Res.*, 4:11-4, 1990

Didry N et al., Antimicrobial activity of some naphtoquinones found in plants, Ann. Pharm. Fr., 44:73-8, 1985

Evans BK et al., Further Studies on the Correlation Between Biological Activity and Solubility of Some Carminatives, J. Pharm. Pharmacol., 27(suppl.):66, 1975

Kasahara T, The anthelmintic action of chenopodium oil, Nipp. Yaku. Zasshi, 52:663-77, 1956 (Chem. Abs. 52:1468b)

Lish PM & Dungan KW, Peristaltic-Stimulating and Fecal-Hydrating Properties of Dioctyl Sodium Sulfosuccinate, Danthron, and Cascara Extracts in the Mouse and Rat, J. Am. Pharm. Assoc., 47:371-5, 1958

Matsui M & Asai M, Analysis of menthone, isomenthone, anethole, and cinnamaldehyde in crude drugs by headspace gas chromatography, Shim. Hyo., 44:219-23, 1987 (Chem. Abs. 108:119050e)

Muller W-U & Leistner E, Aglycones and Glycosides of Oxygenated Naphthalenes and a Glycosyltransferase from Juglans, Phytochem., 17:1739-42, 1978

Nestler T et al., Quantitative determination of bitter-quassinoids of Quassia amara and Picrasma excelsa, Planta Med., 38:204-13, 1980

Nozawa Y, Anthelmintic action of principles of volatile oils. I. Action on pig Ascaris, Sapp. Med. J., 3:48-53, 1952 (Chem. Abs. 50:10928h)

Passet J, Chemical variability within thyme, its manifestations and its significance, Parfums, Cosmet., Aromes, 28:39-42, 1979 (Chem. Abs. 92:72683x)

Phillips RA et al., Cathartics and the Sodium Pump, Nature, 206:1367-8, 1965

Rees WD et al., Treating irritable bowel syndrome with peppermint oil, Brit. Med. J., pp. 835-6, Oct. 6, 1979

Sayed MD et al., A study of the volatile oil and fatty acids of Artemisia absinthium, Bull. Fac. Pharm. (Cairo Univ.),16:85-98, 1977 (Chem. Abs. 92:90953q)

Slepetys J, Essential oil in common wormwood, Polez. Rast. Priblat. Respub. Beloruss., Mater. Nauch. Konf., 2nd, pp. 289-93, 1973 (Chem. Abs. 81:60957z)

Sturdik E et al., Mechanism of antiyeast activity of juglone, a naturally occurring 1,4-naphthoquinone, Biologia (Bratislava),38:343-51, 1983 (Chem. Abs. 99:67412y)

Sugiyama T, The actions of 4-(4-chlorophenylazo)phenol on earthworm and on intestinal parasites of animals, Nipp. Yaku. Zasshi, 56:1054-66, 1960 (Chem. Abs. 55:27651f)

Take Y et al., Role of the Naphthoquinone Moiety in the Biological Activities of Sakyomicin A, J. Antibiot., 39:557-63, 1986

Taylor BA et al., Inhibitory effect of peppermint oil on gastrointestinal smooth muscle, Gut, 24:992, 1983

Valette G et al., Antihelminthic action of the components of essential oils,

Ann. Pharm. Franc., 11:649-53, 1953 (*Chem. Abs.* 48:4181d)

Van den Broucke CO, New pharmacologically important flavonoids of Thymus vulgaris, *World Crops: Prod., Util., Descr.,* 7:271-6, 1982 (*Chem. Abs.* 98:149494v)

Wagner H & Demuth G, Investigations of the anthra glycosides from Rhamnus species, IV. The structure of the cascarosides from Rhamnus purshianus DC, *Z. Naturforsch., B: Anorg. Chem., Org. Chem.,* 31b:267-72, 1976 (*Chem. Abs.* 84:135998m)

Wagner H et al., New constituents of Picrasma excelsa. I., *Planta Med.,* 36:113-8, 1979

Wilbur JM & Sublett KL, Juglone: A Comparison of Natural and Syn thetic Products, *J. Chem. Educat.,* 54:156, 1977

Diuretic and Urinary Antiseptic Formula

Amin AH et al., Berberine sulfate: antimicrobial activity, bioassay, and mode of action, *Can. J. Microbiol.,* 15:1067-76, 1969

Bauer R et al., TLC and HPLC Analysis of Echinacea pallida and E. angustifolia Roots, *Planta Med.,* 54:426-30, 1988

Bauer R et al., Immunological in vivo and in vitro Examinations of Echinacea Extracts, *Arzneim.-Forsch.,* 38:2767-81, 1988

Batyuk V et al., Flavonoids of Solidago virgaurea L. and S. canadensis L. and their pharmacological properties, *Rastit. Resur.,* 24:92-9, 1988 (*Chem. Abs.* 108:201741q)

Beaune A & Balea T, Experimental anti-inflammatory properties of the marshmallow (Althaea officinalis). Potentiation of the topical effect of corticoids, *Therapie,* 21:341-7, 1966 (*Chem. Abs.* 65:1267c)

Britton G & Haslam E, Gallotannins. Part XII. Phenolic Constituents of Arctostaphylos uva-ursi L. Spreng, *J. Chem. Soc.,* pp. 7312-9, 1965

Constantine GH Jr et al., Phytochemical Investigation of Arctostaphylos columbiana Piper and Arctostaphylos patula Greene (Ericaceae), *J. Pharm. Sci.,* 55:1378-82, 1966

Frohne D, Urinary disinfectant activity of bearberry leaf extracts, *Planta Med.,* 18:1-25, 1969

Fuchs L & Iliev V, Isolation of quercitrin from Solidago virga aurea, Solidago serotina, and Solidago canadensis. An old medicinal plant in a new light, *Sci. Pharm.,* 17:128-31, 1949 (*Chem. Abs.* 44:5538d)

Havsteen B, Flavonoids, A Class of Natural Products of High Pharmaco logical Potency, *Biochem. Pharmacol.,* 32:1141-8, 1983

Hocking GM, Echinacea Angustifolia (Cone Flower) As Crude Drug, *Quart. J. Crude Drug Res.,* 5:679-83, 1965

Holopainen M et al., Antimicrobial activity of some Finnish ericaceous plants, *Acta Pharm. Fenn.*, 97:197-202, 1988 (*Chem. Abs.* 111:36508w)

Iwu MM & Ohiri FC, Anti-arthritic triterpenoids of Lonchocarpus cyanescens: benth., *Can. J. Pharm. Sci.*, 15:39-42, 1980

Jahodar L et al., Antimicrobial action of arbutin and the extract from leaves of Arctostaphylos uva-ursi in vitro, *Cesk. Farm.*, 34:174-8, 1985 (*Chem. Abs.*, 103:68188t)

Kitanov G et al., Contents of arbutin in Arctostaphylos uva-ursi (L.) Spreng. from different regions of the Bulgarian People's Republic, *Rastit. Resur.*, 22:425-31, 1986 (*Chem. Abs.* 105:149792d)

Kowalewski Z et al., Antibiotic action of b-ursolic acid, *Arch. Immunol Ther. Exp.*, 24:115-9, 1976

Kreitmair H, Pharmacological trials with some domestic plants, *E. Merck's Jahresber.*, 50:102-10, 1936 (*Chem. Abs.* 31:3149)

Kubo M et al., Pharmacological studies on leaf of Arctostaphylos uva-ursi (L.) Spreng. I. Combined effect of 50% methanolic extract from Arctostaphylos uva-ursi (L.) Spreng. (bearberry leaf) and predniso lone on immuno-inflammation, *Yaku. Zasshi*, 110:59-67, 1990 (*Chem. Abs.* 112:151442c)

Leifertova L et al., Elimination of arbutin from the body, *Rozvoj Farm. Ramci Ved.-Tech. Revoluce, Sb. Prednasek Sjezdu Cesk. Farm. Spol.*, *7th*, pp. 41-3, 1977 (*Chem. Abs.* 93:60998m)

Leifertova I et al., Evaluation of phenolic substances in Arctostaphylos uva ursi. V. Determination of phenolic substances in the aerial parts, *Cesk. Farm.*, 34:415-6, 1985 (*Chem. Abs.* 104:115944u)

Mahajan VM et al., Antimycotic Activity of Berberine Sulphate: An Alkaloid From An Indian Medicinal Herb, *Sabouraudia*, 20:79-81, 1982

Morimoto K et al., Triterpenoid constituents of the leaves of Arctostaphy los uva-ursi, *Muko. Joshi Daig. Kiyo, Yaku. Hen*, 31:41-4, 1983 (*Chem. Abs.* 101:107343v)

Murach M et al., Saponins of genus Solidago. 2. Bayogenin, a sapogenin in Solidago canadensis, *Pharmazie*, 30:619-20, 1975 (*Chem. Abs.* 83:190377n)

Otsuka H et al., Studies on anti-inflammatory agents. II. Anti-inflamma tory constituents from rhizome of Coptis japonica Makino, *Yaku. Zasshi*, 101:883-90, 1981 (*Chem. Abs.* 96:28395p)

Pietta P et al., Identification of flavonoids from Ginkgo biloba L., Anthemis nobilis L. and Equisetum arvense L. by high-performance liquid chromatoography with diode-array UV detection, *J. Chromatogr.*, 553:223-31, 1991

Poptopal'skii AI et al., Antimicrobic and antineoplastic properties of alkaloids of greater celandine and their thiophosphamide derivatives, *Mikrobiol. Zh. (Kiev)*, 37:755-9, 1975 *(Chem. Abs.* 84:84760t)

Suess TR & Stermitz FR, Alkaloids of Mahonia repens with a Brief Review of Previous Work in the Genus Mahonia, *J. Nat. Prod.*, 44:680-7, 1981

Sun D et al., Berberine sulfate blocks adherence of Streptococcus pyogenes to epithelial cells, fibronectin, and hexadecane, *Antimicrob. Agents Chemother.*, 32:1370-4, 1988

Sun D et al., Influence of berberine sulfate on synthesis and expression of Pap fimbrial adhesin in uropathogenic Escherichia coli, *Antimicrob. Agents Chemother.*, 32:1274-7, 1988

Tarle D et al., Equiseta (horsetail plant) - Study of flavonoid and saponin contents, *Farm. Vestn. (Ljubljana)*, 31:303-6, 1980 *(Chem. Abs.* 95:3394d)

Tomoda M et al., Plant mucilages. XVI. Isolation and characterization of a mucous polysaccharide, "Althaea-mucilage O," from roots of Althaea officinalis, *Chem. Pharm. Bull.*, 25:1357-62, 1977

IV BREATHING

Breathe Freely Formula

Abood LG et al., Structure-Activity Studies of Carbamate and Other Esters: Agonists and Antagonists to Nicotine, *Pharmacol. Biochem. Behav.*, 30:403-8, 1988

Anand CL, Treatment of Opium Addiction, *Br. Med. J.*, p. 640, Sep. 11, 1971

Anand CL, Effect of Avena sativa on Cigarette Smoking, *Nature,* 233:496, 1971

Bacon JD et al., Chemosystematics of the Hydrophyllaceae: Flavonoids of Three Species of Eriodictyon, *Biochem. Syst. Ecol.*, 14:591-5, 1986

Connor J et al., The pharmacology of Avena sativa, *J. Pharm. Pharmac.*, 27:92-8, 1975

Hulme A & Bateson MC, Complications of Carbenoxolone Therapy, *Br. Med. J.*, p. 804, Sep. 28, 1974

Jack RAF, Treatment of Opium Addiction, *Br. Med. J.*, p. 48, Oct. 2, 1971

Johnson ND, Flavonoid Aglycones from Eriodictyon californicum Resin and their Implications for Herbivory and UV Screening, *Biochem. Syst. Ecol.*, 11:211-5, 1983

Krochmal A et al., Lobeline content of Lobelia inflata. Structural, Environ mental, and developmental effects, *U.S. Dep. Agr., Forest Serv., Res. Paper, NE,* NE-178, 13 pp., 1970 *(Chem. Abs.* 75:106182z)

London SJ, Clinical Evaluation of a New Lobeline Smoking Deterrent, *Curr. Ther. Res.*, 5:167-75, 1963

McFarland JW, Physical Measures Used in Breaking the Smoking Habit, *Arch. Phys. Med. Rehab.*, p. 323-7, Apr., 1965

Mitscher LA et al., Antimicrobial Agents from Higher Plants. Antimicro bial Isoflavanoids and Related Substances from Glycyrrhiza Glabra L. var. Typica, *J. Nat. Prod.*, 43:259-69, 1980

Mori T et al., Effects of oral administration of glycyrrhizin and its combinations on urine volume and electrolyte metabolism in rats, *Oyo Yak.*, 34:293-301, 1987 (*Chem. Abs.* 108:49307t)

Nishino H et al., Antitumor-promoting activity of glycyrrhetic acid in mouse skin tumor formation induced by 7,12-dimethylbenz[a]anthracene plus teleocidin, *Carcinogen.*, 5:1529-30, 1984

Plakun AL et al., Clinical Factors in Smoking Withdrawal: Preliminary Report, *Am. J. Pub. Health,* 56:434-41, 1966

Pompei R et al., Glycyrrhizic acid inhibits virus growth and inactivates virus particles, *Nature,* 281:690, 1979

Raffalt GJ, Composition for use in weaning persons from tobacco, *Chem. Abs.*, 85:323, 1976 (#182442f)

Reavill C et al., High Affinity Binding of [^{3}H] (-)-Nicotine to Rat Brain Membranes and its Inhibition by Analogues of Nicotine, *Neuropharmacol.*, 27:235-41, 1988

Salle AJ et al., Studies on the Antibacterial Properties of Eriodictyon californicum, *Arch. Biochem Biophys.*, 32:121-3, 1951

Smith MO, Acupuncture and Natural Healing in Drug Detoxification, *Am. J. Acupunct.*, 7:97-106, 1979

Tangri KK et al., Biochemical Study of Anti-Inflammatory and Anti-Arthritic Properties of Glycyrrhetic Acid, *Biochem. Pharmacol.*, 14:1277-81, 1965

Antiviral and Antibacterial Formula

Abe N et al., Interferon Induction by Glycyrrhizin and Glycyrrhetinic Acid in Mice, *Microbiol. Immunol.*, 26:535-9, 1982

Alstat E, Lomatium Dissectum: An Herbal Virucide?, *Complement. Med.*, pp. 32-4, May/June, 1987

Anderson DM & Smith WG, The Antitussive Activity of Glycyrrhetinic Acid and its Derivatives, *J. Pharm. Pharmacol.*, 13:396-404, 1961

Bye RA Jr, Medicinal Plants of the Sierra Madre: Comparative Study of Tarahumara and Mexican Market Plants, *Econ. Bot.*, 40:103-24, 1986

Call TG & Green J, Spasmolytics from Plants. I: Suksdorfin A and Columbianin, *Proc. Mont. Acad. Sci.*, 16:49-51, 1956

Chandler RF et al., Ethnobotany and Phytochemistry of Yarrow, Achillea millefolium, Compositae, *Econ. Bot.*, 36:203-23, 1982

Cohen RA et al., Antiviral Activity of Melissa officinalis (Lemon Balm) Extract, *Proc. Soc. Exp. Biol. Med.,* 117:431-4, 1964

Delaveau P et al., Stimulation of the Phagocytic Activity of R.E.S. by Plant Extracts, *Planta Med.,* 40:49-54, 1980

Delgado G et al., Secondary Metabolites From the Roots of Ligusticum porteri (Umbelliferae). X-ray Structure of Z-6.6',7.3a'-Diligustilide, *Heterocyc.,* 27:1305-12, 1988

Dentali SJ & Hoffmann JJ, Potential Antiinfective Agents from Eriodic tyon angustifolium and Salvia apiana, *Int. J. Pharmacognosy,*30:223-31, 1992

Dikshit A & Husain A, Antifungal action of some essential oils against animal pathogens, *Fitoterapia,* 55:171-6, 1984 *(Chem. Abs.* 102:109670u)

Herrmann EC Jr & Kucera LS, Antiviral Substances in Plants of the Mint Family (Labiatae). II. Nontannin Polyphenol of Melissa officinalis, *Proc. Soc. Exp. Biol. Med.,* 124:869-74, 1967

Herrmann K, The "tannin" in leaves of Labiatae, *Arch. Pharm.,* 293:1043-8, 1960 *(Chem. Abs.* 55:8764b)

Hoerhammer L, Flavone concentration of medicinal plants with regard to their spasmolytic action, *Congr. Sci. Farm., Conf. Comun., 21st, Pisa,* pp. 578-88, 1961 *(Chem. Abs.* 61:3571c)

Hulme A & Bateson MC, Complications of Carbenoxolone Therapy, *Br. Med. J.,* p. 804, Sep. 28, 1974

Hunn ES & French DH, Lomatium: A Key Resource for Columbia Plateau Native Subsistence, *Northwest Sci.,* 55:87-94, 1981

Ko WC et al., Phytochemical studies on spasmolytic constituents of Ligusticum wallichii Franch, *Hua Hsueh,* (3):74-6, 1978 *(Chem. Abs.* 92:37764c)

Kucera LS et al., Antiviral Activities of Extracts of the Lemon Balm Plant, *Ann. N.Y. Acad. Sci.,* 130:474-82, 1965

Kucera LS & Herrmann EC Jr, Antiviral Substances in Plants of the Mint Family (Labiatae). I. Tannin of Melissa officinalis, *Proc. Soc. Exp. Biol. Med.,* 124:865-9, 1967

May G & Willuhn G, Antiviral Activity of Aqueous Extracts from Medicinal Plants in Tissue Cultures, *Arzneim.-Forsch.,* 28:1-7, 1978

Mitscher LA et al., Antimicrobial Agents from Higher Plants. Antimicro bial Isoflavanoids and Related Substances from Glycyrrhiza Glabra L. var. Typica, *J. Nat. Prod.,* 43:259-69, 1980

Mose JR & Lukas G, Studies on the Antibacterial Action of some Ethereal Oils and their Ingredients, *Arzneim.-Forsch.,* 7:687-92, 1957

Pompei R et al., Glycyrrhizic acid inhibits virus growth and inactivates virus particles, *Nature,* 281:690, 1979

Pompei R et al., Antiviral activity of glycyrrhizic acid, *Experientia*, 36:304, 1980

Simoes CMO et al., Preliminary Studies of Antiviral Activity of Triterpenoid Saponins: Relationships Between their Chemical Structure and Antiviral Activity, *Planta Med.*, 56:652-3, 1990

VanWagenen BC & Cardellina JH II, Native American Food and Medicinal Plants 7. Antimicrobial Tetronic Acids from Lomatium dissectum, *Tetrahed.*, 42:1117-22, 1986

VanWagenen BC et al., Native American Food and Medicinal Plants, 8. Water-Soluble Constituents of Lomatium Dissectum, *J. Nat. Prod.*, 51:136-41, 1988

Wagner H Sprinkmeyer L, Pharmacological effect of balm spirit, *Deut. Apoth.-Ztg.*, 113:1159-66, 1973 (*Chem. Abs.* 80:244j)

Cough Relief and Expectorant Formula

Abe N et al., Interferon Induction by Glycyrrhizin and Glycyrrhetinic Acid in Mice, *Microbiol. Immunol.*, 26:535-9, 1982

Albert-Puleo M, Fennel and Anise as Estrogenic Agents, *J. Ethnopharm.*, 2:337-44, 1980

Anderson DM & Smith WG, The Antitussive Activity of Glycyrrhetinic Acid and its Derivatives, *J. Pharm. Pharmacol.*, 13:396-404, 1961

Belkin M et al., Swelling and Vacuolization Induced in Ascites Tumor Cells by Polysaccharides from Higher Plants, *Cancer Res.*, 19:1050-62, 1959

Bennett JP et al., Inhibitory Effects of Natural Flavonoids on Secretion from Mast Cells and Neutrophils, *Arzneim.-Forsch.*, 31:433-7, 1981

Boyd EM & Palmer ME, The Effect of Quillaia, Senega, Squill, Grindelia, Sanguinaria, Chionanthus and Dioscorea upon the Output of Respiratory Tract Fluid, *Acta Pharmacol. Toxicol.*, 2:235-246, 1946

Boyd EM, Expectorants and Respiratory Tract Fluid, *Pharmacol. Rev.*, 6:521-42, 1954

Boyd EM & Sheppard EP, An Autumn-Enhanced Mucotropic Action of Inhaled Terpenes and Related Volatile Agents, *Pharmacol.*, 6:65-80, 1971

Bredeck HE et al., Chemoceptor reflexes in swine, *Am. J. Physiol.*, 201:89-91, 1961

Cahen R, Pharmacologic spectrum of Marrubium vulgare, *C. R. Soc. Biol.*, 164:1467-72, 1970 (*Chem. Abs.* 75:2494m)

Call TG & Green J, Spasmolytics from Plants. I: Suksdorfin A and Columbianin, *Proc. Mont. Acad. Sci.*, 16:49-51, 1956

Cheney RH, Grindeliae Robustae Herba Medicinal Revaluation, *Quart. J. Crude Drug Res.*, 2:169-73, 1962

Greenaway W et al., Flavonoid aglycones identified by gas chromatogra phy-mass spectrometry in bud exudate of Populus balsamifera, *J. Chromatogr.,* 472:393-400, 1989

Guseva EN, Physiological mobility of a respiratory center and the action of respiratory analeptics (lobeline, cytitone, corconium), *Tr. Kuibyshev. Med. Inst.,* 34:37-47, 1965 *(Chem. Abs.* 67:20429h)

Halmagyi D et al., Protective Effect of Lobeline in Experimental Pulmo nary Oedema, *Arch. Int. Pharmacodyn.,* 106:17-27, 1956

Haranath PSRK et al., Acetylcholine and choline in common spices, *Phytother. Res.,* 1:91-2, 1987

Harun J & Labosky P Jr, Chemical Constituents of Five Northeastern Barks, *Wood Fiber Sci.,* 17:275-80, 1985

Karryev MO et al., Some therapeutic properties and phytochemistry of common horehound, *Izv. Akad. Nauk Turkm. SSR, Ser. Biol. Nauk,* (3):86-8, 1976 *(Chem. Abs.* 86:2355u)

Kowalewski Z et al., Action of helenin on microorganisms, *Arch. Immunol. Ther. Exp.,* 24:121-5, 1976

Leshchankina VV & Filatova RN, Seasonal and age-related changes in the yield of underground organs of Inula helenium and its essential oil content, *Prod. Ispol'z Dik. Kul't. Rast.,* pp. 114-22, 1983 *(Chem. Abs.* 102:93090s)

Mitscher LA et al., Antimicrobial Agents from Higher Plants. Antimicro bial Isoflavanoids and Related Substances from Glycyrrhiza Glabra L. Var. Typica, *J. Nat. Prod.,* 43:259-69, 1980

Pompei R et al., Glycyrrhizic acid inhibits virus growth and inactivates virus particles, *Nature,* 281:690, 1979

Pompei R et al., Antiviral activity of glycyrrhizic acid, *Experientia,* 36:304, 1980

Saxe TG, Toxicity of Medicinal Herbal Preparations, *AFP,* 35:135-42, 1987

Simon IS & Shostenko YV, Lobeline determination in plant material, *Farm. Zh. (Kiev),* 14:51-3, 1959 *(Chem. Abs.* 60:371c)

Subba MS et al., Antimicrobial Action of Citrus Oils, *J. Food Sci.,* 32:225-7, 1967

Tamas M & Popescu H, Determination of volatile components of Inulae radix, fluid extract, *Farmacia (Bucharest),* 30:169-72, 1982 *(Chem. Abs.* 98:77992f)

Timmermann BN et al., Quantitative Variation of Grindelane Diterpene Acids in 20 Species of North American Grindelia, *Biochem. Syst. Ecol.,* 15:401-10, 1987

VanWagenen BC & Cardellina JH II, Native American Food and Medici nal Plants 7. Antimicrobial Tetronic Acids from Lomatium dissectum, *Tetrahed.,* 42:1117-22, 1986

VanWagenen BC et al., Native American Food and Medicinal Plants, 8.

Water-Soluble Constituents of Lomatium Dissectum, *J. Nat. Prod.*, 51:136-41, 1988

Zukerman I, Effect of Oxidized d-Limonene on Micro-organisms, *Nature,* 168:517, 1951

V CIRCULATION

Heart Tonic Formula

Ammon HPE & Handel M, Crataegus, Toxicology and Pharmacology, *Planta Med.,* 43:105-20, 209-39, 313-22, 1981

Bauer U, 6-Month Double-blind Randomised Clinical Trial of Ginkgo biloba Extract versus Placebo in Two Parallel Groups in Patients Suffering from Peripheral Arterial Insufficiency, *Arzneim.-Forsch,* 34:716-20, 1984

Brown SD et al., Cactus Alkaloids, *Phytochem.,* 7:2031-6, 1968

Chatterjee SS & Gabard B, Studies on the Mechanism of Action of an Extract of Ginkgo biloba, a Drug Used for Treatment of Ischemic Vascular Diseases, *Arch. Pharmacol.,* 320:R52, 1982

Chung KF et al., Effect of a Ginkgolide Mixture (BN 52063) in Antagonising Skin and Platelet Responses to Platelet Activating Factor in Man, *Lancet,* pp. 248-51, Jan. 31, 1987

Congora C et al., Isolation and identification of two mono-C-glucosylluteolins and of the di-C-substituted 6,8-diglucosylluteolin from the leafy stalks of Passiflora incarnata L., *Helv. Chim. Acta,* 69:251-3, 1986 (*Chem. Abs.* 104:183298m)

Feroz H & Khare AK, Preliminary Pharmacological Investigation on Cactus grandiflorus, *Indian Drugs,* 20:113, 1982

Guendjev Z, Experimental Myocardial Infarction of the Rat and Stimula tion of the Revascularization by the Flavonoid Drug Crataemon, *Arzneim.- Forsch.,* 27:1576-9, 1977

Guillon JM et al., Effects of Ginkgo biloba extract on various in vitro and in vivo models of experimental myocardial ischaemia, *Presse Med.,* 15:1516-9, 1986

Iwamoto et al., Klinische Wirkung von Crataegutt bei Herzerkrankungen ischamischer und/oder hypertensiver Genese. Eine multizentrische Doppelblindstudie, *Planta Med.,* 42:1-15, 1981

Kandziora J, Demonstration of the Crataegutt effect in patients with perfusion disorders of the coronary arteries. EKG findings with the effort test, *Munch. Med. Wochens.,* 111:295-300, 1969

Kartnig T et al., Investigations on the Procyanidin and Flavonoid contents of Crataegus monogyna-Drugs, *Sci. Pharm.,* 55:95-100, 1987

Lamaison JL & Carnat A, Content of principal flavonoids of the flowers and leaves of Crataegus monogyna Jacq. and Crataegus laevigata

(Poiret) DC. (Rosaceae), *Pharm. Acta Helv.,* 65:315-20, 1990 (*Chem. Abs.* 114:78654h)

Lewak S et al., Polymeric flavans of hawthorn leaves (Crataegus oxyacantha), *Rocz. Chem.,* 44:1733-9, 1970 (*Chem. Abs.* 74:108111d)

Manolov P, Pharmacologic characteristics of the preparation Crataemon, *Suvrem. Med.,* 22:20-3, 1971 (*Chem. Abs.* 77:444n)

Mavers WH & Hensel H, Changes in Local Myocardial Blood Flow Following Oral Administration of a Crataegus Extract to Non-anesthetized Dogs, *Arzneim.-Forsch.,* 24:783-5, 1974

Menghini A & Mancini LA, TLC Determination of Flavonoid Accumula tion in Clonal Populations of Passiflora incarnata L., *Pharm. Res. Comm.,* 20(Supp.):113-6, 1988

Occhiuto F et al., Comparative study on the cardiovascular activity of young shoots, leaves and flowers of Crataegus oxyacantha L., *Plant. Med. Phytother.,* 20:37-51, 52-63, 1986

Occhiuto F et al., Comparative Haemodynamic Effects of the Flavonoids Rhoifolin and Vitexin in the Dog, *Phytother. Res.,* 4:118-20, 1990

Occhiuto F et al., Comparative Antiarrhythmic and Anti-ischaemic Activity of some Flavones in the Guinea-pig and Rat, *Phytother. Res.,* 5:9-14, 1991

Peter H, Vasoactivity of Ginkgo biloba preparations, *Conf. Hung. Ther. Invest. Pharmacol., Soc. Pharmacol. Hung., 4th,* pp. 177-81, 1966 (*Chem. Abs.* 722:11142k)

Petershofer-Halbmayer H et al., Isolation of Hordenine ("Cactine") from Selenicereus grandiflorus (L.) Britt. & Rose and Selenicereus pteranthus (Link & Otto) Britt. & Rose, *Sci. Pharm.,* 50:29-34, 1982

Pietta P et al., Identification of flavonoids from Ginkgo biloba L., Anthemis nobilis L. and Equisetum arvense L. by high-performance liquid chromatography with diode-array UV detection, *J. Chromatogr.,* 553:223-231, 1991

Prabhakar MC et al., Pharmacological Investigations on Vitexin, *Planta Med.,* 43:396-403, 1981

Quercia V et al., Identification and determination of vitexin and isovitexin in Passiflora incarnata extracts, *J. Chromatogr.,* 161:396-402, 1978

Rewerski W & Lewak S, Some Pharmacological Properties of Flavan Polymers Isolated from Hawthorn (Crataegus oxyacantha), *Arzneim.-Forsch.,* 17:490-1, 1967

Rewerski W et al., Some Pharmacological Properties of Oligomeric Procyanidin Isolated from Hawthorn (Crataegus oxyacantha), *Arzneim.-Forsch.,* 21:886-8, 1971

Roddewig C & Hensel H, Reaction of local myocardial blood flow in non-anesthetized dogs and anesthetized cats to the oral and parenteral administration of a Crateagus fraction (oligomere procyanidines), *Arzneim.-Forsch.,* 27:1407-10, 1977

Tanniere M & Rochette L, Direct effects of platelet activating factor (PAF) on cardiac function in isolated guinea pig heart, *Drug Dev. Res.,* 11:177-86, 1987

Taskov M et al., Some cardiovascular effects of crataemon, *Farmatsiya (Sofia),* 27:30-4, 1977 (*Chem. Abs.* 87:161754k)

Trunzler G & Schuler E, Comparative Studies on the Effects of a Crataegus Extract, Digitoxin, Digoxin and g-Strophanthin in the Isolated Heart of Homoiothermals, *Arzneim.-Forsch.,* 12:198, 1962

VanBeek TA et al, Determination of ginkgolides and bilobalide in Ginkgo biloba leaves and phytopharmaceuticals, *J. Chromatogr.,* 543:375-87, 1991

Vargha A, Treatment of the coronary syndrome and cardiac failure with Adenylocrat and Adenylocrat-Digoxin, *Munch. Med. Wochens.,* 112:2247-50, 1970

Vorberg G, Ginkgo Biloba Extract (GBE): A long-Term Study of Chronic Cerebral Insufficiency in Geriatric Patients, *Clin. Trials J.,* 22:149-57, 1985

Wagner H & Grevel J, New Cardioactive Drugs II, Detection and Isolation of Cardiotonic Amines with Ionpair-HPLC, *Planta Med.,* 44:36-40, 1982

Wagner H & Grevel, Cardioactive Drugs IV. Cardiotonic Amines from Crataegus oxyacantha, *Planta Med.,* 45:98-101, 1982

Balanced Blood Formula

Allen FM, Blueberry leaf extract, *J.A.M.A.,* 89:1577-81, 1927

Baj A et al., Qualitative and Quantitative Evaluation of Vaccinium myrtillus Anthocyanins by High-Resolution Gas Chromatography and High-Performance Liquid Chromatography, *J. Chromatogr.,* 279:365-72, 1983

Bettini V et al., Interactions between Vaccimium myrtillus anthocyanosides and serotonin on splenic artery smooth muscle, *Fitoterapia,* 55:201-8, 1984

Bettini V et al., Effects of Vaccinium myrtillus anthocyanosides on vascular smooth muscle, *Fitoterapia,* 55:265-72, 1984

Bettini V et al., Mechanical responses of isolated coronary arteries to barium in the presence of Vaccinium myrtillus anthocyanosides, *Fitoterapia,* 56:3-10, 1985

Bever BO & Zahnd GR, Plants with Oral Hypoglycaemic Action, *Quart. J. Crude Drug Res.,*17:139-196, 1979

Cignarella A et al., Hypolipidemic Activity of Vaccinium myrtillus Leaves on a New Model of Genetically Hyperlipidemic Rat, *Planta Med.,* 58 (suppl. 1):A581-2, 1992

Detre Z et al., Studies on vascular permeability in hypertension: action of anthocyanosides, *Clin. Physiol. Biochem.,* 4:143-9, 1986

Edgars NK, Blueberry in diabetes, *Drug Cosmetic Ind.,* 35:479-80, 1934 (*Chem. Abs.* 29:7579)

Farnsworth NR & Segelman AB, Hypoglycemic Plants, *Tile & Till,* 57:52-6, 1971

Friedrich H & Schonert J, Hydroxyflavans from Leaves and Fruits of Vaccinium myrtillus L., *Arch. Pharmaz.,* 106:611-5, 1973

Gomez-Serranillos Fernandez M et al., Effects on in vitro platelet aggregation of Vaccimium myrtillus L. anthocyanosides, *An. R. Acad. Farm.,* 49:79-90, 1983 (*Chem. Abs.* 99:16344v)

Ichikawa K et al., The Ca^{2+} Antagonist Activity of Lignans, *Chem. Pharm. Bull.,* 34:3514-7, 1986

Lapinina LO & Sisoeva TF, Investigation of some plants to determine their sugar-lowering action, *Farmatsevt. Zh. (Kiev),* 19:52-8, 1964 (*Chem. Abs.* 66:1451e)

Large RG & Brocklesby HN, A hypoglycemic substance from the roots of the devil's club (Fatsia horrica), *Can. Med. Assoc, J.,* 39:32-5, 1938

Lietti A et al., Studies on Vaccinium myrtillus anthocyanosides I. Vasoprotective and antiinflammatory activity, *Arzneim.-Forsch.,* 26:829-32, 1976

Lietti A & Forni G, Studies on Vaccinium myrtillus anthocyanosides II. Aspects of anthocyanins pharmacokinetics in the rat, *Arzneim.-Forsch.,* 26:832-5, 1976

Luntz GRWN, Insulin substitutes, *Guy's Hosp. Gaz.,* 54:285-8, 1940 (*Chem. Abs.* 35:3333)

Mishkinsky J et al., Hypoglycaemic Effect of Trigonelline, *Lancet,* pp. 1311-2, Dec. 16, 1967

Morazzoni P & Magistretti MJ, Effects of Vaccinium myrtillus anthocyanosides on prostacyclin-like activity in rat arterial tissue, *Fitoterapia,* 57:11-14, 1986

Piccoli LJ et al., A Pharmacologic Study of Devil's Club Root (Fatsia Horrida), *J. Am. Pharm. Assoc.,* 29:11-12, 1940

Racz-Kotilla E et al., The Action of Taraxacum officinale Extracts on the Body Weight and Diuresis of Laboratory Animals, *Planta Med.,* 26:212-7, 1974

Ramstad E, Chemical Investigation of Vaccimium myrtillus L., *J. Am. Pharm. Assoc.,* 43:236-40, 1954

Ribes G et al., Effects of Fenugreek Seeds on Endocrine Pancreatic Secretions in Dogs, *Ann. Nutr. Metab.,* 28:37-43, 1984

Ribes G et al., Hypocholesterolaemic and Hypotriglyceridaemic Effects of

Subfractions from Fenugreek Seeds in Alloxan Diabetic Dogs, *Phytother. Res.*, 1:38-43, 1987

Robert AM et al., Action of Anthocyanosides of Vaccinium myrtillis on the Permeability of the Blood Brain Barrier, *J. Med.*, 8:321-32, 1977

Sevin R & Cuendet JF, Effets d'une association d'anthocyanosides de myrtille et de b-carotene sure la resistance capillaire des diabetiques, *Ophthalmologica*, 152:109-117, 1966

Shani (Mishkinsky) J et al., Hypoglycaemic Effect of Trigonella Foenum Graecum and Lupinus Termis (Leguminosae) Seeds and their Major Alkaloids in Alloxan-Diabetic and Normal Rats, *Arch. Int. Pharmacodyn.*, 210:27-37, 1974

Sharma RD et al., Hypolipidaemic Effect of Fenugreek Seeds. A Clinical Study, *Phytother. Res.*, 5:145-7, 1991

Stuhr ET & Henry FB, The root bark of Fasia horrida, *Pharm. Arch.*, 15:9-15, 1944 *(Chem. Abs.* 38:4092)

Susnik F, The present state of knowledge about the medicinal plant Taraxacum officinale Weber, *Med. Razgl.*, 21:323-8, 1982

Takeda S et al., Kidney disorder-treating agents containing guaiaretic acid, meso-dihydroguaiaretic acid, arctiin, arctigenine, or asarinin, *Chem. Abs.*, 113:401, 1990 (#103446f)

Valette G et al., Hypocholesterolaemic Effect of Fenugreek Seeds in Dogs, *Atheroscler.*, 50:105-11, 1984

Yamanouchi S et al., Constituents of the fruit of Arctuim lappa, *Yaku. Azsshi*, 96:1492-3, 1976 *(Chem. Abs.* 86:136299n)

Zaragoza F et al., Comparative studies on the antiaggregating effects of anthocyanosides and other agents, *Arch. Farmacol. Toxicol.*, 11:183-8, 1985 *(Chem. Abs.* 104:141972w)

Venous Tonic Formula

Boido A et al., N-Substituted derivatives of rosmaricine, *Studi Sassar., Sez. 2*, 53:383-93, 1975 *(Chem. Abs.* 88:69046d)

Brieskorn CH et al., Determination of ursolic acid and ethereal oils in Labiatae of pharmaceutical and nutritional importance, *Arch. Pharm.*, 285:290-6, 1952 *(Chem. Abs.* 47:7164f)

Brieskorn CH et al., Flavones of rosemary leaves, *Deut. Lebensm.-Rundsch.*, 69:245-6, 1973

Detre Z et al., Studies on vascular permeability in hypertension: action of anthocyanosides, *Clin. Physiol. Biochem.*, 4:143-9, 1986

Fish F & Waterman PG, Alkaloids in the bark of Zanthoxylum clava-herculis, *J. Pharm. Pharmac.*, 25(Suppl.):115P-6P, 1973

Friedrich H Schonert J, Hydroxyflavans from Leaves and Fruits of Vaccimium myrtillus L., *Arch. Pharm.*, 106:611-5, 1973

Frohne D, Urinary disinfectant activity of bearberry leaf extracts, *Planta Med.,* 18:1-25, 1969

Gerhardt U & Schroeter A, Rosmarinic acid - a naturally occurring antioxidant in spices, *Fleischwirt.,* 63:1628-30, 1983 *(Chem. Abs.* 100:33386s)

Gomez-Serranillos Fernandez M et al., Effects on in vitro platelet aggrega tion of Vaccinium myrtillus L. anthocyanosides, *An. R. Acad. Farm.,* 49:79-90, 1983 *(Chem. Abs.* 99:16344v)

Gracza L & Ruff P, Occurrence and analysis of phenylpropane derivatives, V. Rosmarinic acid in pharmacopeial drugs and its determination by HPLC, *Arch. Pharm. (Weinheim, Ger.),* 317:339-45, 1984 *(Chem. Abs.* 100:215600q)

Grigorescu M et al., Ointment with venotropic action, *Chem. Abs.,* 92:387, 1980 (#64774n)

Jamstyn H, The active constituents of Hamamelis virginiana, *Parfuem. Kosmetik,* 45:335-7, 1964 *(Chem. Abs.* 62:12323f)

Kellner W & Kober W, The Possibility of using Ethereal Oils for the Disinfection of Rooms, *Arzneim.-Forsch.,* 5:224-9, 1955

Kowalewski Z et al., Action of helenin on microorganisms, *Arch. Immunol. Ther. Exp.,* 24:121-5, 1976

Lenfeld J et al., Antiinflammatory Activity of Quaternary Benzophenanthridine Alkaloiids from Chelidonium majus, *Planta Med.,* 43:161-5, 1981

Lietti A et al., Studies on Vaccinium myrtillus anthocyanosides I. Vasoprotective and antiinflammatory activity, *Arzneim.-Forsch.,* 26:829-32, 1976

Maffei Facino R et al., Mass spectrometry for the direct analysis of gallotannins, *Chim. Oggi,* (7-8):48-52, 1985 *(Chem. Abs.* 104:31147y)

Morazzoni P & Magistretti MJ, Effects of Vaccinium myrtillus anthocyanosides on prostacyclin-like activity in rat arterial tissue, *Fitoterapia,* 57:11-14, 1986 *(Chem. Abs.* 105:54290z)

Powell CE & Chen KK, The Pharmacological Action of Chelerythrine, *J. Am. Pharm. Assoc.,* 44:196-9, 1955

Ramstad E, Chemical Investigation of Vaccinium myrtillus L., *J. Am. Pharm. Assoc.,* 43:236-40, 1954

Rao KV & Davies R, The Ichthyotoxic Principles of Zanthoxylum Clava-Herculis, *J. Nat. Prod.,* 49:340-2, 1986

Robert AM et al., Action of Anthocyanosides of Vaccinium myrtillis on the Permeability of the Blood Brain Barrier, *J. Med.,* 8:321-32, 1977

Sendra J et al., Chromatographic analysis of flavonoids and triterpenes in folium rosmarini, *Diss. Pharm. Pharmacol.,* 21:185-91, 1969

Ulrichova J et al., Inhibition of Acetylcholinesterase Activity by some Isoquinoline Alkaloids, *Planta Med.,* 48:111-5, 1983

Wenkert E et al., Chemical artifacts from the family Labiatae, *J. Org. Chem.*, 30:2931-4, 1965

Zaragoza F et al., Comparative studies on the antiaggregating effects of anthocyanosides and other agents, *Arch. Farmacol. Toxicol.*, 11:183-8, 1985 (*Chem. Abs.* 104:141972w)

VI MIND & MOOD

Mental Energy Formula

Abramova ZI et al., Stimulation of catechol amines and serotonin circula tion caused by Eleutherococcus and dibazole, *Lek. Sredstva Dal'nego Vostoka*, 11:106-8, 1972 (*Chem. Abs.* 82:38660w)

Afanas'eva TN & Lebkova NP, Effect of Eleutherococcus on subcellular heart structures in experimental myocardial infarction, *Byull. Eksp. Biol. Med.*, 103:212-5, 1987 (*Chem. Abs.* 106:188712t)

Anand CL, Treatment of Opium Addiction, *Br. Med. J.*, p. 640, Sep. 11, 1971

Brekhman II & Dardymov IV, Pharmacological Investigation of Glyco sides from Ginseng and Eleutherococcus, *Lloydia*, 32:46-51, 1969

Chowdhury AKA et al., Biological activity of the alcohol extract and the glycosides of Hydrocotile asiatica Linn., *J. Bangladesh Acad. Sci.*, 11:75-82, 1987 (*Chem. Abs.* 107:108725g)

Connor J et al., The pharmacology of Avena sativa, *J. Pharm. Pharmac.*, 27:92-8, 1975

Dardymov IV, Gonadotropic action of Eleutherococcus glycosides, *Lek. Sredstva Dal'nego Vostoka*, 11:60-5, 1972 (*Chem. Abs.* 82:51571n)

Dardymov IV et al., Insulinlike action of eleutherosides from the roots of Eleutherococcus senticosus, *Rastit. Resur.*, 14:86-9, 1978 (*Chem. Abs.* 88:115363e)

Del Vecchio A et al., Effects of Centella asiatica on biosynthetic activity in cultured fibroblasts, *Farmaco, Ed. Prat.*, 39:355-64, 1984 (*Chem. Abs.* 101:204298s)

De Souza NJ et al., Preparation of 2,3,23-trihydroxyuro-12-ene and its derivatives as serotonergic receptor antagonists, *Chem. Abs.*, 115:426, 1991 (#189738d)

Doly M et al., Effect of Ginkgo biloba extract on the electrophysiology of the isolated diabetic rat retina, *Presse Med.*, 15:1480-3, 1986

Etienne A et al., Mechanism of action of Ginkgo biloba extract on experimental cerebral oedema, *Presse Med.*, 15:1506-10, 1986

Filaretov AA et al., Effect of adaptogens on the activity of the pituitary-adrenocortical system in rats, *Byull. Eksp. Biol. Med.*, 101:573-4, 1986 (*Chem. Abs.* 105:54415u)

Galushkina LP et al., Effects of the eleutherosides, phenols, and polysaccharides of Eleutherococcus on adaptation and responsiveness of the
central nervous system in ischemia, *Farmatsiya (Moscow)*, 39:59-63,
1990 (*Chem. Abs.* 112:210887b)

Gebner B et al., Study of the Long-Term Action of a Ginkgo biloba
Extract on Vigilance and Mental Performance as Determined by
Means of Quantitative Pharmaco-EEG and Psychometric Measure
ments, *Arzneim.-Forsch.*, 35:1459-65, 1985

Golotin VG et al., Effect of ionol and Eleutherococcus extract on alter
ations in rat hypophyseal-adrenal system under conditions of stress,
Vopr. Med. Khim., 35:35-7, 1989 (*Chem. Abs.* 110:128610f)

Hindmarch I, Activity of Ginkgo biloba extract on short term memory,
Presse Med., 15:1592-4, 1986

Kaemmerer K & Fink J, Studies on the extract of eleutheroccoccus with
regard to trophanabole reactions in the rat, *Prakt. Tierarzt*, 61:748-60,
1980 (*Chem. Abs.* 94:3119x)

Karcher L et al., Effect of an extract of Ginkgo biloba on rat brain energy
metabolism in hypoxia, *Naunyn-Schmied. Arch. Pharmacol.*, 327:31-
5, 1984

Krieglstein J et al., Influence of an Extract of Ginkgo biloba on Cerebral
Blood Flow and Metabolism, *Life Sci.*, 39:2327-34, 1986

Lamour Y et al., Effects of ginkgolide B and ginkgo biloba extract on local
cerebral glucose utilization in the awake adult rat, *Drug Dev. Res.*,
23:219-25, 1991

Leonova EV, Effect of Eleutherococcus and dibazole on the pathological
and compensatory response of an animal during experimental brain
ischemia, *Aktual. Probl. Tior. Klin. Med.*, pp. 262-4, 1975 (*Chem.
Abs.* 87:95994k)

Leonova EV & Bregman IG, Effect of adaptogens on work capacity and
resistance to experimental brain ischemia, *Zdravookhr. Beloruss.*,
(3):13-6, 1979 (*Chem. Abs.* 90:197767t)

Le Poncin Lafitte M et al., Effects of Ginkgo Biloba on Changes Induced
by Quantitative Cerebral Microembolization in Rats, *Arch. Int.
Pharmacodyn.*, 243:236-44, 1980

Marina TF, Comparative effects of extracts of Panax, Leuzea, and
Eleutherococcus on the electroencephalograms of rabbits,
Stimulyatory Tsentl. Nerv. Sist., pp. 24-30, 1966 (*Chem. Abs.*
66:93852e)

Mikaelyan EM et al., Regulation of some biochemical indexes of blood by
Eleutherococcus glycosides during acute stress, *Zh. Eksp. Klin. Med.*,
26:421-6, 1986 (*Chem. Abs.* 107:70777k)

Morier-Teissier E et al., Changes in the levels of catecholamines,
indolamines and their metabolites in the brain of mice and rat

following acute and chronic administration of a Ginkgo biloba leaf extract, *Biog. Amines,* 4:351-8, 1987 *(Chem. Abs.* 108:161196g)

Nishiyama N et al., Effect of Eleutherococcus senticosus and its compo nents on sex- and learning-behaviors and tyrosine hydroxylase activities of adrenal gland and hypothalamic regions in chronic stressed mice, *Shoya. Zasshi,* 39:238-42, 1985 *(Chem. Abs.* 104:102465p)

Pearce PT et al., Panax ginseng and Eleutherococcus senticosus extracts - in vitro studies on binding to steroid receptors, *Endocrinol. Jpn.,* 29:567-73, 1982 *(Chem. Abs.* 98:137807m)

Pidoux B, Effects of Ginkgo biloba extract on functional activity of the brain, *Presse Med.,* 15:1588-91, 1986

Pointel JP et al., Titrated Extract of Centella Asiatica (TECA) in the Treatment of Venous Insufficiency of the Lower Limbs, *Angiology,* 38:46-50, 1987

Poizot A & Dumez D, Modification of the healing kinetics after iterative exeresis in the rat. Action of titrated extract of Centella asiatica (TECA) on duration of healing, *C. R. Hebd. Seances Acad. Sci., Ser. D,* 286:789-92, 1978 *(Chem. Abs.* 88:183073k)

Rai GS et al., A double-blind, placebo controlled study of Ginkgo biloba extract ("Tanakan') in elderly out-patients with mild to moderate memory impairment, *Curr. Med. Res. Opin.,* 12:350-5, 1991

Sadykov SB et al., Effect of Eleutherococcus senticosus extract on the T-system immune response during stress, *Zdravookhr. Daz.,* (11):52-5, 1987 *(Chem. Abs.* 108:68519e)

Saratikov AS, Central nervous system stimulants of plant origin, *Stimulyatory Tsent. Nerv. Sist.,* pp. 3-23, 1966 *(Chem. Abs.* 70:10069p)

Schaffler K & Reeh PW, Double-blind Study of the Hypoxia-Protective Effect of a Standardised Ginkgo bilobae Preparation after Repeated Administration in Healthy Volunteers, *Arzneim.-Forsch.,* 35:1283-8, 1985

Singh B & Rastogi RP, Chemical Examination of Centella asiatica Linn - III. Constitution of Brahmic Acid, *Phytochem.,* 7:1385-93, 1968

Spinnewyn B et al., Effects of Ginkgo biloba extract on a cerebral is chaemia model in gerbils, *Presse Med.,* 15:1511-5, 1986

Taillandier J et al., Ginkgo biloba extract in the treatment of cerebral disorders due to aging, *Presse Med.,* 15:1583-7, 1986

Takasugi N et al., Effect of Eleutherococcus senticosus and its components on rectal temperature, body and grip tones, motor coordination, and exploratory and spontaneous movements in acute stressed mice, *Shoya. Zasshi,* 39:232-7, 1985 *(Chem. Abs.* 104:102464n)

Tauritis A, Hypophysis-adrenal system in technological stress and its prevention in industrial animal husbandry, *LLA Raksti,* 247:87-93, 1988 (*Chem. Abs.* 111:17899h)

Upadhyay SC et al., Total glycoside content and antistress activity of Indian and Mauritius Centella asiatica - a comparison, *Indian Drugs,* 28:388-9, 1991 (*Chem. Abs.* 115:198456n)

Vogel HG et al., Effect of terpenoids isolated from Centella asiatica on granuloma tissue, *Acta Ther.,* 16:285-98, 1990 (*Chem. Abs.* 114:221326k)

Vorberg G, Ginkgo biloba Extract (GBE): A Long-Term Study of Chronic Cerebral Infufficiency in Geriatric Patients, *Clin. Trials J.,* 22:149-57, 1985

Soothing Sedative Formula

Achterrath-Tuckermann U et al., Pharmacological Investigations with Compounds of Chamomile V. Investigations on the Spasmolytic Effect of Compounds of Chamomile and Kamillosan on the Isolated Guinea Pig Ileum, *Planta Med.,* 39:38-50, 1980

Albert-Puleo M, Fennel and Anise as Estrogenic Agents, *J. Ehtnopharmacol.,* 2:337-44, 1980

Aoyagi N et al., Studies on Passiflora incarnata Dry Extract. I. Isolation of Maltol and Pharmacological Action of Maltol and Ethyl Maltol, *Chem. Pharm. Bull.,* 22:1008-1013, 1974

Balderer G & Borbely AA, Effect of valerian on human sleep, *Psychopharm.,* 87:406-9, 1985

Boeters U, On Treatment of Control Disorders of the Autonomic Nervous System with Valepotriaten (Valmane), *Munch. Med. Wochen.,* 111:1873-6, 1969

Caujolle F et al., Spasmolytic action of Hop (Humulus lupulus), *Agressologie,* 10:405-10, 1969 (*Chem. Abs.* 72:41267x)

von Eickstedt KW & Rahman S, Psychopharmacologic Effects of Valepotriates, *Arzneim.-Forsch.,* 19:316-9, 1969

von Eickstedt KW, Influence of Valepotriates on the Effect of Alcohol, *Arzneim.-Forsch.,* 19:995-7, 1969

Fink C et al., Effects of Valtrate on the EEG of the Isolated Perfused Rat Brain, *Arzneim.-Forsch.,* 34:170-3, 1984

Hansel R & Wohlfart R, Narcotic Action of 2-Methyl-3-butene-2-ol Contained in the Exhalation of Hops, *Z. Naturforsch.,* 35:1096-7, 1980

Hansel R et al., The Sedative-Hypnotic Principle of Hops 3. Communication: Contents of 2-Methyl-3-butene-2-ol in Hops and Hop Preparations, *Planta Med.,* 45:224-8, 1982

Haranath PSRK et al., Acetylcholine and choline in common spices,
    Phytother. Res., 1:91-2, 1987
Hartley RD & Fawcett CH, Identification of Volatile, Water-Soluble
    Compounds from Hops (Humulus Lupulus L.), *Phytochem.,* 7:1395-
    1400, 1968
Hazelhoff B et al., Antispasmotic Effects of Valeriana Compounds: An in-
    Vivo and in-Vitro Study on the Guinea-Pig Ileum, *Arch. Int.
    Pharmacodyn.,* 257:274-87, 1982
Hendriks H et al., Pharmacological Screening of Valerenal and some other
    other Components of Essential Oil of Valeriana officinalis, *Planta
    Med.,* 42:62-8, 1981
Hendriks H et al., Central Nervous Depressant Activity of Valerenic Acid
    in the Mouse, *Planta Med.,* (1):28, 1985
Herisset A et al., Flavonoids of Roman camomille (Anthemis nobilis),
    simple variety, *Plant. Med. Phytother.,* 7:234-40, 1973 *(Chem. Abs.*
    81:1257y)
Holzl J & Fink C, Effect of Valepotriates on Locomotor Activity of Mice,
    Arzneim.-Forsch., 34:44-7, 1984
Jakovlev V et al., Pharmacological Investigations with Compounds of
    Chamomile VI. Investigations on the Antiphlogistic Effects of
    Chamazulene and Matricine, *Planta Med.,* 49:67-73, 1983
Leathwood PD et al., Aqueous Extract of Valerian Root (Valeriana
    officinalis L.) Improves Sleep Quality im Man, *Pharm. Biochem
    Behav.,* 17:65-71, 1982
Lessin AW et al., The Central Stimulant Properties of Some Substituted
    Indolylalkylamines and b-Carbolines and their Activities as Inhibitors
    of Monoamine Oxidase and the Uptake of 5-Hydroxytryptamine, *Br.
    J. Pharmacol.,* 29:70-9, 1967
Lutomski J & Wrocinski T, Pharmacodynamic properties of Passiflora
    incarnata preparations. The effect of alkaloid and flavonoid compo-
    nents on pharmacodynamic properties of the raw material, *Biul. Inst.
    Roslin Leczn.,* 6:176-84, 1960 *(Chem. Abs.* 55:6785e)
Menghini A & Mancini LA, TLC Determination of Flavonoid Accumula-
    tion in Clonal Populations of Passiflora incarnata L., *Pharmacol. Res.
    Comm.,* 20(Suppl. V):113-6, 1988
Nano GM et al., Genus Anthemis. I., *Essenze Deriv. Agrum.,* 43:107-14,
    1973 *(Chem. Abs.* 80:143045f)
Nano GM et al., Botanical and chemical studies on Anthemis nobilis L.
    and some of its cultivars, *Ess.enzeDeriv. Agrum.,* 46:171-5, 1976
    (Chem. Abs. 86:177153d)
Petkov VD et al., Pharmacological studies on a mixture of valepotriates
    isolated from Valeriana officinalis, *Dokl. Bolg. Akad. Nauk,* 27:1007-
    10, 1974 *(Chem. Abs.* 82:51636n)

Petkov V & Manolov P, Pharmacological Studies on Substances of Plant
    Origin with Coronary Dilatating and Antiarrhythmic Action, *Comp.*
    Med. East West, 6:123-30, 1978

Prabhakar MC et al., Pharmacological Investigations on Vitexin, *Planta*
    Med., 43:396-403, 1981

Prokopenko AP et al., Pharmacological and chemical properties of hops
    Humulus lupulus, *Farm. Zh. (Kiev),* (1):28-30, 1986 *(Chem. Abs.*
    104:155777y)

Stern P & Milin R, Antiallergic and Antiphlogistic Effects of Azulene
    Substances, *Arzneim.-Forsch.,* 6:445-450, 1956

Wagner H & Jurcic K, On the Spasmolytic Activity of Valeriana Extracts,
    Planta Med., 37:84-6, 1979

Wohlfart R et al., The Sedative-hypnotic Principle of Hops 4. Communica-
    tion: Pharmacology of 2-Methyl-3-buten-2-ol, *Planta Med.,* 48:120-3,
    1983

Wohlfart R et al., Detection of sedative-hypnotic hop constituents V.
    Degradation of humulones and lupulones to 2-methyl-3-buten-2-ol, a
    hop constituent possessing sedative-hypnotic activity, *Arch. Pharm.*
    (Weinheim, Ger.), 316:132-7, 1983 *(Chem. Abs.* 98:132234n)

Children's Calming Elixir Formula

Achterrath-Tuckermann U et al., Pharmacological Investigations with
    Compounds of Chamomile V. Investigations on the Spasmolytic
    Effect of Compounds of Chamomile and Kamillosan on the Isolated
    Guinea Pig Ileum, *Planta Med.,* 39:38-50, 1980

Baslas RK & Saxena S, Chromatographic analysis of dementholized
    essential oil of Mentha piperita, *Indian J. Phys. Nat. Sci.,* 4:31-2, 1984
    (Chem. Abs. 101:188008q)

Brieskorn CH et al., Determination of ursolic acid and ethereal oils in
    Labiatae of pharmaceutical and nutritional importance, *Arch. Pharm.,*
    285:290-6, 1952 *(Chem. Abs.* 47:7164f)

Dikshit A & Husain A, Antifungal action of some essential oils against
    animal pathogens, *Fitoterapia,* 55:171-6, 1984 *(Chem. Abs.*
    102:109670u)

Evans BK et al., Further Studies on the Correlation Between Biological
    Activity and Solubility of Some Carminatives, *J. Pharm. Pharmacol.,*
    27(Suppl.):66P, 1975

Forster HB et al., Antispasmodic Effects of Some Medicinal Plants, *Planta*
    Med., 40:309-19, 1980

Gerhardt U & Schroeter A, Rosmarinic acid - a naturally occurring
    antioxidant in spices, *Fleischwirt.,* 63:1628-30, 1983 *(Chem. Abs.*

100:33386s)

Haensel R & Kussmaul M, Two triterpenes from elder blossoms, *Arch. Pharm. (Weinheim, Ger.)*, 308:790-2, 1975 *(Chem. Abs.* 84:56476m)

Haragsimova L, Effect produced in vitro on Bacillus larvae by inhibitors of plant origin, *Ved. Prace Vzykum. Ustavu Vcelar Skebo,*(3):13-52, 1963 *(Chem. Abs.* 65:1075h)

Harney JW et al., Behavioral and Toxicological Studies of Cyclopentanoid Monoterpenes From Nepeta cataria, *Lloydia,* 41:367-74, 1978

Hatch RC, Effect of drugs on catnip (Nepeta cataria)-induced pleasure behavior in cats, *Amer. J. Vet. Res.,* 33:143-55, 1972 *(Chem. Abs.* 76:149004f)

Herrmann K, The "tannin" in leaves of Labiatae, *Arch. Pharm.,* 293:1043-8, 1960 *(Chem. Abs.* 55:8764b)

Herrmann EC Jr & Kucera LS, Antiviral Substances in Plants of the Mint Family (Labiatae). II. Nontannin Polyphenol of Melissa officinalis, *Proc. Soc. Exp. Biol. Med.,* 124:869-74, 1967

Herrmann EC Jr & Kucera LS, Antiviral Substances in Plants of the Mint Family (Labiatae). III. Peppermint (Mentha piperita) and other Mint Plants, *Proc. Soc. Exp. Biol. Med.,* 124:874-8, 1967

Hilal SH et al., Investigation of the volatile oil of Hyssopus officinalis L., *Egypt. J. Pharm. Sci.,* 19:177-84, 1978 *(Chem. Abs.* 94:205411x)

Hilal SH et al., Study of the flavonoid content of Hyssopus officinalis l., *Egypt. J. Pharm. Sci.,* 20:271-8, 1979 *(Chem. Abs.* 98:31407r)

Hoffmann BG & Lunder LT, Flavonoids from Mentha piperita Leaves, *Planta Med.,* 50:361, 1984

Iwu MM & Ohiri FC, Anti-arthritic triterpenoids of Lonchocarpus cyanescens: benth., *Can. J. Pharm. Sci.,* 15:39-42, 1980

Jakovlev V et al., Pharmacological Investigations with Compounds of Chamomile VI. Investigations on the Antiphlogistic Effects of Chamazulene and Matricine, *Planta Med.,* 49:67-73, 1983

Herisset A et al., Flavonoids of Roman camomille (Anthemis nobilis), simple variety, *Plant. Med. Phytother.,* 7:234-40, 1973 *(Chem. Abs.* 81:1257y)

Kalashnikova NA & Gerashchenko GI, Antiphlogistic activity of several flavonoids, *Aktual. Vopr. Farm.,* 2:353-4, 1974 *(Chem. Abs.* 84:99346m)

Kucera LS & Herrmann EC Jr, Antiviral Substances in Plants of the Mint Family (Labiatae). I. Tannin of Melissa officinalis, *Proc. Soc. Exp. Biol. Med.,* 124:865-9, 1967

Leifertova I et al., Substances contained in flowers and fruit of Sambucus, during the growth period, *Acta Fac. Pharm., Univ. Comeniana,* 20:57-82, 1971 *(Chem. Abs.* 77:16587x)

Liao C, Studies on the antispasmodic effects of kaempferol, *Kuo Li Chung-kuo I yao Yen Chiu So Yen Chiu Pao Kao,* pp. 79-94, 1984 *(Chem. Abs.* 102:89964n)

McElvain SM & Eisenbraun EJ, The Constituents of the Volatile Oil of Catnip. III. The Structure of Nepetalic Acid and Related Compounds, *J. Am. Chem. Soc.,* 77:1599-1605, 1955

Nano GM et al., Genus Anthemis. I. *Ess. Deriv. Agrum.,* 43:107-14, 1973 *(Chem. Abs.* 80:143045f)

Nano GM et al., Botanical and chemical research on Anthemis nobilis and some of its cultivars, *Essenze Deriv. Agrum.,*46:171-5, 1976 *(Chem. Abs.* 86:177153d))

Radu A et al., Comparative study of flavones in indigenous elder flowers (Sambucus nigra L., S. ebulus L., S. racemosa L.), *Farmacia (Bucharest),* 24:9-15, 1976 *(Chem. Abs.* 85:74954r)

Regnier FE et al., Studies on the Composition of the Essential Oils of Three Nepeta Species, *Phytochem.,* 6:1281-9, 1967

Richter W & Willuhn G, Data on the Constituents of Sambucus nigra L. III. Determination of ursol and oleanol acids, amyrin and sterol contents from Sambuci DAB 7 flowers, *Pharm. Ztg.,* 122:1567-71, 1977 *(Chem. Abs.* 87:189344a)

Roshchin YV & Gerashchenko GI, Anti-inflammatory activity of some flavonoids, *Vopr. Farm. Dal'nem Vostoke,* 1:134-5, 1973 *(Chem. Abs.* 83:37682p)

Stern P & Milin R, Antiallergic and Antiphlogistic Effects of Azulene Substances, *Arzneim.-Forsch.,* 6:445-50, 1956

Tagawa M & Murai F, A New Iridoid Glucoside, Nepetolglucosylester from Nepeta cataria, *Planta Med.,* 39:144-7, 1980

Thieme H & Kitze C, Occurrence of flavonoids in Melissa officinalis, *Pharmazie,* 28:69-70, 1973 *(Chem. Abs.* 78:108197u)

Wagner H & Sprinkmeyer L, Pharmacological effect of balm spirit, *Deut. Apoth.-Ztg.,* 113:1159-66, 1973 *(Chem. Abs.* 80:244j)

Willuhn G & Richter W, The constituents of Sambucus nigra. II. The lipophilic components of the flowers, *Planta Med.,* 31:328-43, 1977 *(Chem. Abs.* 90:51444p)

Zaletova NI et al., Preparation of some derivatives of ursolic acid and their antimicrobial activity, *Khim.-Farm. Zh.,* 20:568-71, 1986 *(Chem. Abs.* 106:18867e)

VII WOMEN & MEN

Premenstrual Ease Formula

Altmann G, Effect of gonadotropic substances and sex hormones of vertebrates on the honeybee ovary, *Z. Bienenforsch.*, 6:135-6, 1963 (*Chem. Abs.* 65:65:12513g)

Aradhana et al., Diosgenin - a growth stimulator of mammary gland of ovariectomized mouse, *Indian J. Exp. Biol.*, 30:367-70, 1992 (*Chem. Abs.* 116:248828d)

Barlow RB & McLeod LJ, Some studies on cytisine and its methylated derivatives, *Br. J. Pharmac.*, 35:161-74, 1969

Belic I et al., A biologically active substance from Vitex agnus-castus seeds, *Vestnik Sloven. kemi. drustva,* 5:63-7, 1958 (*Chem. Abs.* 54:19959a)

Belic I et al., Constituents of Vitex agnus castus seeds. I. Casticin, *J. Chem. Soc.,* pp. 2523-5, 1961

Cayen MN et al., Studies on the disposition of diosgenin in rats, dogs, monkeys and man, *Atheroscler.*, 33:71-87, 1979

Cha L et al., Antiarrhythmic effect of Angelica sinensis root, tetrandrine and Sophora flavescens root, *Yao Hsueh T'ung Pao,* 16:53-4, 1981 (*Chem. Abs.* 95:126047a)

Che C-T, Phytochemical Investigations of Aristolochia indica L. and Caulophyllum thalictroides (L.) Michaux, *Diss. Abs. Int.*, 43:1049B, 1982

Chen Y et al., Analysis of the composition of Angelica sinensis - determination of the essential oil composition by capillary column GC/MS, *Gao. Xue. Hua. Xue.*, 5:125-8, 1984 (*Chem. Abs.* 100:188755k)

DeCapite L, Histology, anatomy, and antibiotic properties of Vitex agnuscastus, *Ann. Fac. Agr. Univ. Studi Perugia,* 22:109-26, 1967 (*Chem. Abs.* 71:73980)

Farnsworth NR, The plant kingdom - supplier of steroids, *Tile Till,* 53:55-7, 1967

Ferguson HC & Edwards LD, A Pharmacological Study of a Crystalline Glycoside of Caulophyllum thalictroides, *J. Am. Pharm. Assoc.,* 43:16-21, 1954

Flom MS et al., Isolation and Characterization of Alkaloids from Caulophyllum thalictroides, *J. Pharm. Sci.,* 56:1515-7, 1967

Jochle W, Menses-Inducing Drugs: Their Role in Antique, Medieval and Renaissance Gynecology and Birth Control, *Contracept.*, 10:425-37, 1974

Juarez-Oropeza MA et al., In vivo and in vitro studies of hypocholesterolemic effects of diosgenin in rats, *Int. J. Biochem.,* 19:679-83, 1987

Karryev MO, Study of some essential oils from Turkmen plants, *Izv. Akad. Nauk Turkm. SSR, Ser. Biol. Nauk,* (5):11-16, 1966 (*Chem. Abs.* 66:118808k)

Ko W-C et al., Alkylphthalides isolated from Ligusticum wallichii Franch and their in vitro inhibitory effect on rat uterine contraction induced by prostaglandin F$_{2a}$, *T'ai-wan I Hsueh Hui Tsa Chih*, 76:669-77, 1977 (*Chem. Abs.* 88:130721p)

Lin M et al., Studies on the chemical constituents of Angelica sinensis, *Yao Hsueh Hsueh Pao*, 14:529-34, 1979 (*Chem. Abs.* 92:177412m)

Liu Z et al., Antiasthmatic effect of n-butenyl phthalide from Dang Gui and some other synthetic derivatives of phthalide, *Zhongcaoyao*, 13:17-21, 1982 (*Chem. Abs.* 97:174444r)

McShefferty J & Stenlake JB, Caulosapogenin and its Identity with Hederagenin, *J. Chem. Soc.*, pp. 2314-6, 1956

Mishurova SS et al., Essential oil of Vitex agnus castus L., its fractional composition and antimicrobial activity, *Rastit. Resur.*, 22:526-30, 1986 (*Chem. Abs.* 106:116495b)

Ozaki Y & Ma JP, Inhibitory effects of tetramethylpyrazine and ferulic acid on spontaneous movement of rat uterus in situ, *Chem. Pharm. Bull.*, 38:1620-3, 1990

Sliutz G et al., Agnus Castus Extracts Inhibit Prolactic Secretion of Rat Pituitary Cells, *Horm. Met. Res.*, 25:253-5, 1993

Spiegel EA & Wycis HT, Anticonvulsant effects of steroids, *J. Lab. Clin. Med.*, 30:947-53, 1945

Sung C-P et al., Effect of Extracts of Angelica polymorpha on Reaginic Antibody Production, *J. Nat. Prod.*, 45:398-406, 1982

Tao J et al., Studies on the antiasthmatic effect of ligustilide of Dang Gui, Angelica sinensis (Oliv.) Diels, *Xaoxue Xuebao*, 19:561-5, 1984 (*Chem. Abs.* 101:183841q)

Terasawa K et al., Chemical and clinical evaluation of crude drugs derived from Angelica acutilobae and A. sinensis, *Fitoterapia*, 56:201-8, 1985 (*Chem. Abs.* 104:141747b)

Tewari PV et al., Experimental Study on Estrogenic Activity of Diosgenin Isolated from Costus speciosus Sm., *Indian J. Pharm.*, 35:35-6, 1973

Tsay R, Radix Angelicae Sinensis - Tang Kuei, *New Chin. Med.*, pp. 36-41, June, 1973

Wall ME et al., Steroidal Sapogenins XII. Survey of Plants for Steroidal Sapogenins and Other Constituents, *J. Am. Pharm. Assoc.*, 43:503-5, 1954

Wall ME et al., Steroidal Sapogenins XXV. Survey of Plants for Steroidal Sapogenins and Other Constituents, *J. Am. Pharm. Assoc.*, 44:438-40, 1955

Wollenweber E & Mann K, Flavonols from fruits of Vitex agnus castus, *Planta Med.*, 48:126-7, 1983

Yin Z-Z et al., Effect of Dang-Gui (Angelica sinensis) and its ingredient ferulic acid on rat platelet aggregation and release of 5-HT, *Yao Hsueh Hsueh Pao*, (6):321-6, 1980 (*Chem. Abs.* 94:266g)

Phytoestrogen Aid Formula

Albert-Puleo M, Fennel and Anise as Estrogenic Agents, *J. Ethnopharmacol.*, 2:337-44, 1980

Anguelakova M et al., Cutaneous effect of phyto-estrogen compounds of certain medicinal drugs, *Parfums, Cosmet., Savons Fr.*, 2:555-7, 1972 (*Chem. Abs.* 78:62061q)

Arustamova FA, Hypotensive effect of Leonurus cardiaca on animals in experimental chronic hypertension, *Izv. Akad. Nauk Arm. SSR, Biol. Nauki*, 16:47-52, 1963 (*Chem. Abs.* 60:6101e)

Bickoff EM et al., Relative Potencies of Several Estrogen-Like Compounds Found in Forages, *Agric. Fd. Chem.*, 10:410-2, 1962

Bickoff EM et al., Isolation of Coumestrol and Other Phenolics from Alfalfa by Countercurrent Distribution, *J. Pharm. Sci.*, 53:1496-9, 1964

Bravo L et al., Pharmacodynamic study of hops (Humulus lupulus), *Ars Pharm.*, 12:421-5, 1971 (*Chem. Abs.* 79:133139e)

Buzogany K & Cucu V, Comparattive study between the species Leonurus cardiaca L. and Leonurus quinquelobatus Gilib. Part II. Iridoids, *Clujul Med.*, 56:385-8, 1983 (*Chem. Abs.* 100:65051v)

Cabo Torres J & Bravo Diaz L, Pharmacodynamic study of hops (Humulus lupulus) IV. Antioxytocic activity, *Ars Pharm.*, 12:191-201, 1971 (*Chem. Abs.* 77:29359z)

Cheng EW et al., Estrogenic Activity of some Naturally Occurring Isoflavones, *N.Y. Acad. Sci.*, 61:652-9, 1955

Chury J, Uber den Phytoostrogengehalt einiger Pflanzen, *Experientia*, 16:194-5, 1960

Chury J, The antigonadotrophic action of lucerne: Medicago sativa, *Ann. Endocrin., Paris*, 29:699-702, 1968

Costello CH & Lynn EV, Estrogenic Substances from Plants: I. Glycyrrhiza, *J. Am. Pharm. Assoc.*, 39:177-80, 1950

Elakovich SD & Hampton JM, Analysis of Coumestrol, a Phytoestrogen, in Alfalfa Tablets Sold for Human Consumption, *J. Agric. Food Chem.*, 32:173-5, 1984

Erspamer V, Pharmacology of Leonurus cardiaca and Leonurus marrubiastrum L., *Arch. intern. pharmacodynamie*, 76:132-52, 1948 (*Chem. Abs.* 42:8961h)

Farnsworth NR et al., Potential Value of Plants as Sources of New Antifertility Agents II, *J. Pharm. Sci.*, 64:717-54, 1975

Fenselau C & Talalay P, Is Oestrogenic Activity Present in Hops?, *Fd. Cosmet. Tosicol.*, 11:597-603, 1973

Folman Y & Pope GS, Effect of Norethisterone Acetate, Dimethylstilboestrol, Genistein and Coumestrol on Uptake of [³H]Oestradiol by Uterus, Vagina and Skeletal Muscle of Immature Mice, *J. Endocr.*, 44:213-8, 1969

Gizycki H, The influence of medicinal plants on the female genital system-experiments on white rats and mice with Cimicifuga racemosa, *Z. ges. exptl. Med.*, 113:635-44, 1944 (*Chem. Abs.* 44:759a)

Guggolz J et al., Detection of Daidzein, Formononetin, Genistein, and Biochanin A in Forages, *Agricult. Fd. Chem.*, 9:330-2, 1961

Gulubov AZ & Chervenkova VB, Structure of alkaloids from Leonurus cardiaca, *Nauch. Tr. Vissh. Pedagog. Inst., Plovdiv, Mat., Fiz., Khim., Biol.*, 8:129-32, 1970 (*Chem. Abs.* 74:39177r)

Isaev I & Bojadzieva M, Obtaining galenic and neogalenic preparations and experiments for the isolation of an active substance from Leonurus cardiaca, *Nauchni. Tr. Visshiya Med. Inst., Sofiya*, 37:145-52, 1960 (*Chem. Abs.* 58:4373h)

Jarry H & Harnischfeger G, Studies on the endocrine effects of constituents from Cimicifuga racemosa. 1. Influence on the serum concentration of pituitary hormones in ovariectomized rats, *Planta Med.*, (1);46-9, 1985 (*Chem. Abs.* 102:215969h)

Jarry H et al., Studies on the endocrine effects of the contents of Cimicifuga racemosa. 2. In vitro binding of compounds to estrogen receptors, *Planta Med.*, (4):316-9, 1985 (*Chem. Abs.* 103:200749h)

Kartnig T et al., Flavonoid-O-Glycosides from the Herbs of Leonurus cardiaca, *J. Nat. Prod.*, 48:494-507, 1985

Knuckles BE et al., Coumestrol Content of Fractions Obtained during Wet Processing of Alfalfa, *J. Agric. Food Chem.*, 24:1177-80, 1976

Kumagai A et al., Effect of Glycyrrhizin on Estrogen Action, *Endocrinol. Japon.*, 14:34-8, 1967

Kumai A et al., Extraction of biologically active substances from hop, *Nipp. Naibun. Gak. Zasshi*, 60:1202-13, 1984 (*Chem. Abs.* 102:21265e)

Kumai A & Okamoto R, Extraction of the Hormonal Substance from Hop, *Toxicol. Lett.*, 21:203-7, 1984

Leavitt WW & Meismer DM, Sexual Development altered by Non-steroidal Oestrogens, *Nature*, 218:181-2, 1968

Martin PM et al., Phytoestrogen Interaction with Estrogen Receptors in Human Breast Cancer Cells, *Endocrinol.*, 103:1860-7, 1978

McKendree CA et al., Mechanics of pain and treatment of dysmenorrhea, *Clin. Med. Surg.*, 44:536-40, 1937 (*Chem. Abs.* 32:3823)

Newsome FE & Kitts WD, Effects of alfalfa consumption on estrogen levels in ewes, *Can. J. Anim. Sci.*, 57:531-5, 1977

Noteboom WD & Gorski J, Estrogenic Effect of Genistein and
    Coumestrol Diacetate, *Endocrinol.*, 7:736-9, 1963
Reiners W, 7-Hydroxy-4'-methoxy-isoflavon (Formononetin) aus
    Sussholzwurzel. Uber Inhaltsstoffe der Sussholzwurzel. II,
        Experiencia,22:359, 1966
Saitoh T & Shibata S, Chemical Studies on the Oriental Plant Drugs.
    XXII.[1] Some New Constituents of Licorice Root. (2)[2] Glycyrol, 5-
    O-Methylglycyrol and Isoglycyrol, *Chem. Pharm. Bull.*, 17:729-34,
    1969
Senatore F et al., Sterols from Leonurus cardiaca L. growing in different
    geographical areas, *Herba Pol.*, 37:3-7, 1991 (*Chem. Abs.*
    116:170207d)
Sharaf A & Goma N, Phytoestrogens and their Antagonism to Progester
    one and Testosterone, *J. Endocrin.*, 31:289-90, 1965
Shutt DA, Interaction of Genistein with Oestradiol in the Reproductive
    Tract of the Ovariectomized Mouse, *J. Endocrin.*, 37:231-2, 1967
Shutt DA & Cox RI, Steroid and Phyto-Oestrogen Binding to Sheep
    Uterine Receptors in Vitro, *J. Endocr.*, 52:299-310, 1972
Wash LK & Bernard JD, Licorice-induced Pseudoaldosteronism, *Am. J.
    Hosp. Pharm.*, 32:73-4, 1975
Weinges K et al., Natural products from medinical plants. XVIII. Isolation
    and structure elucidation of a new C_{15}-iridoid glucoside from
    Leonurus cardiaca, *Justus Liebigs Ann. Chem.*, (4):566-72, 1973
    (*Chem. Abs.* 79:75831m)

Prostate Tonic Formula

Albert-Puleo M, Mythobotany, Pharmacology, and Chemistry of Thujone-
    Containing Plants and Derivatives, *Econ. Bot.*, 32:65-74, 1978
Bauer R et al., Immunological in vivo and in vitro Examinations of
    Echinacea Extracts, *Arzneim.-Forsch.*, 38:276-81, 1988
Bauer R et al., TLC and HPLC Analysis of Echinacea pallida and E.
    angustifolia Roots, *Planta Med.*, 54:426-30, 1988
Bauer R et al., Alkamides from the Roots of Echinacea angustifolia,
    Phytochem., 28:505-8, 1989
Belaiche P & Lievoux O, Clinical Studies on the Palliative Treatment of
    Prostatic Adenoma with Extract of Urtica Root, *Phytother. Res.*,
    5:267-9, 1991
Brilery M et al., Permixon, a new Treatment for Benign Prostatic Hyper-
    plasia, Acts Directly at the Cytosolic Androgen Receptor in Rat
    Prostate, *Br. J. Pharmac.*, 79:327P, 1983

Butruille D & Dominguez XA, Fouquierol and isofouquierol, two new triterpenes of the dammarane series, *Tetrahedron Lett.*, (8):639-42, 1974 (*Chem. Abs.* 81:37666v)

Butruille D & Alvarez E, Biogenetic interpretation of the presence of dammarenediol in the roots of Fouquiera splendens, *Rev. Latinoagm. Quim.*, 7:96-7, 1976 (*Chem. Abs.* 85:119520q)

Carilla E et al., Binding of Permixon, a New Treatment for Prostatic Benign Hyperplasia, to the Cytosolic Androgen Receptor in the Rat Prostate, *J. Steroid Biochem.*, 20:521-3, 1984

Champault G et al., A double-blind trial of an extract of the plant Serenoa repens in benign prostatic hyperplasia, *Br. J. Clin. Pharmac.*, 18:461-2, 1984

Chaurasia N & Wichtl M, Sterols and Steryl Glycosides from Urtica dioica, *J. Nat. Prod.*, 50:881-5, 1987

DiSilverio F et al., Evidence that Serenoa repens extract displays an antiestrogenic activity in prostatic tissue of benign prostatic hypertrophy patients, *Eur. Urol.*, 21:309-14, 1992

Elghamry MI & Hansel R, Activity and Isolated Phytoestrogen of Shrub Palmetto Fruits (Serenoa repens Small), a New Estrogenic Plant, *Experientia*, 25:828-9, 1969

El-Sheikh MM et al., The effect of Permixon on androgen receptors, *Obstet. Gyn. Scand.*, 67:397-9, 1988

Frohne D, Urinary disinfectant activity of bearberry leaf extracts, *Planta Med.*, 18:1-25, 1969 (*Chem. Abs.* 72:41331p)

Halls CMM & Warnhoff EW, The Constitution of Ocotillol., *Chem. Ind.*, (51):1986, 1963

Hatinguais P et al., Composition of the hexane extract from Serenoa repens Bartram fruits, *Trav. Soc. Pharm. Montpellier*, 41:253-62, 1981 (*Chem. Abs.* 99:10736c)

Hocking GM, Echinacea angustifolia (Cone Flower) as Crude Drug, *Quart. J. Crude Drug Res.*, 5:679-83, 1965

Hofstetter A & Eisenberger F, Spamso-Urogenin, a new drug for the treatment of diseases of the lower urinary tract and of the male adnexa, *Munch. Med. Wochens.*, 110:619-23, 1968

Dvorakova V, Antimicrobial action of arbutin and the extract from leaves of Arctostaphylos uva-ursi in vitro, *Cesk. Farm.*, 34:174-8, 1985 (*Chem. Abs.* 103:68188t)

Jensen SR & Nielsen BJ, Iridoid Glucosides in Fouquieriaceae, *Phytochem.*, 21:1623-9, 1982

Jommi G et al., Constituents of the lipophilic extract of the fruits of Serenoa repens (Bar.) Small, *Gazz. Chim. Ital.*, 118:823-6, 1988 (*Chem. Abs.* 110:209328x)

Jommi G et al., Alcohols isolated from lipophilic Serenoa repens extracts and their use for the treatment of prostate pathologies, *Chem. Abs.*, 111:394, 1989 (#84073x)

Kellner W & Kober W, The Possibility of using Etherial Oils for the Disinfection of Rooms, *Arzneim.-Forsch.*, 5:224-9, 1955

Leifertova I et al., Elimination of arbutin from the body, *Rozvoj Farm. Ramci Ved.-Tech. Revoluce, Sb. Prednasek Sjezdu Cesk. Farm. Spol.*, *7th*, pp. 41-3, 1979 (*Chem. Abs.* 93:60998m)

Le Moal MA & Truffa-Bachi P, Urtica dioica agglutinin, a new mitogen for murine T lymphocytes: unaltered interleukin 1 production but late interleukin-2-mediated proliferation, *Cell. Immunol.*, 115:24-35, 1988 (*Chem. Abs.* 109:91026w)

Poehland BL et al., In vitro Antiviral Activity of Dammar Resin Triterpenoids, *J. Nat. Prod.*, 50:706-13, 1987

von Rudloff E, Gas-Liquid Chromatography of Terpenes Part IV. The Analysis of the Volatile oil of the Leaves of Eastern White Cedar, *Can. J. Chem.*, 39:1200-5, 1961

Schoepflin G et al., b-Sitosterol as a possible hormone of sabal fruits, *Planta Med.*, 14:402-7, 1966 (*Chem. Abs.* 66:44265g)

Shnyakina GP et al., Arbutin content in the leaves of some plants grown at Dal'nyi Vostok, *Rastit. Resur.*, 17:568-71, 1981 (*Chem. Abs.* 96:3668s)

Smirnoff WA, Effects of Volatile Substances Released by Foliage of Abies balsamea, *J. Invertebrate Pathol.*, 19:32-5, 1972

Sultan C et al., Inhibition of Androgen Metabolism and Binding by a Liposterolic Extract of "Serenoa repens B" in Human Foreskin Fibroblasts, *J. Steroid Biochem.*, 20:515-9, 1984

Takeda S et al., Pharmacological studies on iridoid compounds. II. Relationship between structures and choleretic actions of iridoid compounds, *J. Pharmacobio-Dyn.*, 3:485-92, 1980 (*Chem. Abs.* 94:150017r)

Tarayre JP et al., Anti-edematous action of an hexane extract from Serenoa repens Bartr. drupes, *Ann. Pharmaceutiques franc.*, 41:559-70, 1983

Van Damme IJM et al., The Urtica dioica agglutinin is a complex mixture of isolectins, *Plant Physiol.*, 86:598-601, 1988 (*Chem. Abs.* 108:147213d)

Voaden DJ & Jacobson M, Tumor Inhibitors. 3. Identification and Synthesis of an Oncolytic Hydrocarbon from American Coneflower Roots, *J. Med. Chem.*, 15:619-23, 1972

Vomel T, Influence of a Vegetable Immune Stimulant on Phagocytosis of Erythrocytes by the Reticulohistiocytary System of Isolated Perfused Rat Liver, *Arzneim.-Forsch.*, 35:1437-40, 1985

Walker M, Serenoa repens Extract (Saw Palmetto) Relief for Benign Prostatic Hypertrophy (BPH), *Townsend Lett. Doct.*, 91/92:107-10, 1991

Warnhoff EW & Halls CMM, Desert Plant Constituents II. Ocotillol: an Intermediate in the Oxidation of Hydroxy Isooctenyl Side Chains, *Can. J. Chem.*, 43:3311-21, 1965

VIII ACHES & PAINS

Analgesic and Antispasmodic Formula

Aurousseau M et al., Recherches sur quelques proprietes pharmacodynamiques du Piscidia erythrina L. (Legumineuses), *Ann. Pharm. Franc.*, 23:251-7, 1965

Auxence EG, A Pharmacognostic Study of Piscidia Erythrina, *Econ. Bot.*, 7:270-84, 1953

Connell DW & Sutherland MD, A Re-examination of Gingerol, Shogaol, and Zingerone, the Pungent Principles of Ginger (Zingiber officinale Roscoe), *Aust. J. Chem.*, 22:1033-43, 1969

Costello CH & Butler CL, An Investigation of Piscidia Erythrina (Jamaica Dogwood), *J. Am. Pharm. Assoc.*, 37:89-96, 1948

Della Loggia R et al., Isoflavones as Spasmolytic Principles of Piscidia erythrina, *Plant Flav. Biol.Med.*, 2:365-8, 1988

Flynn DL et al., Inhibition of Human Neutrophil 5-Lipoxygenase Activity by Gingerdione, Shogaol, Capsaicin and Related Pungent Compounds, *Prostagl. Leukotr. Med.*, 24:195-8, 1986

Furgiuele AR et al., Central Activity of Aqueous Extracts of Piper methysticum (Kava), *J. Pharm. Sci.*, 54:247-52, 1965

Genazzani E & Sorrentino L, Vascular Action of Acteina: Active Constituent of Actaea racemosa L., *Nature*, 194:544-5, 1962

Haensel R & Lazar J, Kava pyrones. Composition of Piper methysticum rhizomes in plant derived sedatives, *Dtsch. Apoth. Ztg.*, 125:2056-8, 1985 (*Chem. Abs.* 104:74869c)

Huang Q et al., Anti-5-hydroxytryptamine$_3$ Effect of Galanolactone, diterpenoid Isolated from Ginger, *Chem. Pharm. Bull.*, 39:397-9, 1991

Keller F & Klohs MW, A Review of the Chemistry and Pharmacology of the Constituents of Piper Methysticum, *Lloydia*, 26:1-15, 1963

Kiuchi F et al., Inhibitors of Prostaglandin Biosynthesis from Ginger, *Chem. Pharm. Bull.*, 30:754-7, 1982

Kiuchi F et al., Inhibition of Prostaglandin Biosynthesis by the Constituents of Medicinal Plants, *Chem. Pharm. Bull.*, 31:3391-6, 1983

Kretzschmar R & Meyer HJ, Comparative studies on the anticonvulsive activity of pyrone compounds from Piper methysticum, *Arch. Int. Pharmacodyn. Ther.*, 177:261-77, 1969 (*Chem. Abs.* 72:30057c)

Kretzschmar R et al., Spasmolytic activity of aryl substituted a-pyrones and aqueous extracts of Piper methysticum, *Arch. Int. Pharmacodyn. Ther.,* 180:475-91, 1969 *(Chem. Abs.* 72:20254a)

Macht DI & Cook HM, A Pharmacological Note on Cimicifuga, *J. Am. Pharm. Assoc.,* 21:324-30, 1932

Meyer HJ & May HU, Local anesthetic properties of natural kava pyrones, *Klin. Wochschr.,* 42:407, 1964 *(Chem. Abs.* 61:9932c)

Meyer HJ & Kretzschmar R, Kawa pyrones: a new group of components in central muscle relaxing agents of the mephenesin type, *Klin. Wochschr.,* 44:902-3, 1966 *(Chem. Abs.* 65:12750g)

Meyer HJ, Pharmacology of kava, *Ethnopharmacol. Search Psychoact. Drugs, [Proc. Symp.],* pp. 133-40, 1979 *(Chem. Abs.* 92:121862r)

Monache FD et al., Two Isoflavones from Piscidia erythrina, *Phytochem.,* 23:2945-7, 1984

Moore JA & Eng S, Some New Constituents of Piscidia erythrina L., *J. Am. Chem. Soc.,* 78:395-8, 1956

Mustafa T & Srivastava KC, Ginger (Zingiber officinale) in Migraine Headache, *J. Ethnopharm.,* 29:267-73, 1990

O'Hara MJ et al., Preliminary Characterization of Aqueous Extracts of Piper methysticum (Kava, Kawa Kawa), *J. Pharm. Sci.,* 54:1021-5, 1965

Panizzi L & Corsano S, Actein, *Atti Accad. Nazl. Lincei., Rend., Classe Sci. Fis., mat. Nat.,* 32:601-5, 1962 *(Chem. Abs.* 58:12814e)

Piancatelli G, New triterpenes from Actaea racemosa. IV., *Gazz. Chim. Ital.,* 101:139-48, 1971 *(Chem. Abs.* 75:59763c)

Redaelli C & Santaniello E, Major Isoflavonoids of the Jamaican Dogwood Piscidia erythrina, *Phytochem.,* 23:2976-7, 1984

Schindler H, Die Inhaltsstoffe von Heilpflanzen und Prufungsmethoden fur pflanzliche Tinkturen, *Arzneim.-Forsch.,* 2:547- 9, 1952

Schwarz JSP et al., The Extractives of Piscidia erythrina L. - I The Constitution of Ichthynone, *Tetrahed.,* 20:1317-30, 1964

Srivastava KC, Effect of Onion and Ginger Consumption on Platelet Thromboxane Production in Humans, *Prostagl. Leukotri. Ess. Fatty Acids,* 35:183-5, 1989

Srivastava KC & Mustafa T, Ginger (Zingiber officinale) and Rheumatic Disorders, *Med. Hypothes.,* 29:25-8, 1989

Yamahara J et al., Active Components of Ginger Exhibiting Antiserotonergic Action, *Phytother. Res.,* 3:70-1, 1989

Anti-inflammatory Formula

Backer RC et al., A Phytochemical Investigation of Yucca schottii (Lilliaceae), *J. Pharm. Sci.,* 61:1665-6, 1972

Bennett JP et al., Inhibitory Effects of Natural Flavonoids on Secretion from Mast Cells and Neutrophils, *Arzneim.-Forsch.*, 31:433-7, 1981

Benoit PS et al., Biological and Phytochemical Evaluation of Plants. XIV. Antiinflammatory Evaluation of 163 Species of Plants, *Lloydia*, 39:160-71, 1976

Besora C, Taraxacum officinale, Weber, *Circ. Farm.*, 32:641-3, 1974

Bingham R et al., Yucca Plant Saponin in the Management of Arthritis, *J. Appl. Nutrit.*, 27:45-51, 1975

Bingham R et al., Yucca Plant Saponin in the Treatment of Hypertension and Hypercholesterolemia, *J. Appl. Nutrit.*, 30:127-36, 1978

Bohm K, Studies on the Choleretic Action of some Drugs, *Arzneim.-Forsch.*, 9:376-8, 1959

Burrows S & Simpson JCE, The Triterpene Group. Part IV. The Triterpene Alcohols of Taraxacum Root, *J. Chem Soc.*, pp. 2042-7, 1938

Chaturvedi AK et al., Anti-inflammatory and Anticonvulsant Properties of Some Natural Plant Triterpenoids, *Pharm. Res. Comm.*, 8:199-210, 1976

Della-Loggia R et al., Anti-inflammatory activity of benzopyrones that are inhibitors of cyclo- and lipo-oxygenase, *Pharmacol. Res. Commun.*, 20(Suppl. 5):91-4, 1988

Eichler O & Koch C, On the Antiphlogistic, Analgetic, and Spasmolytic Effects of Harpagosid a Glycoside from the Root of Harpagophytum procumbens DC, *Arzneim.-Forsch.*, 20:107-9, 1970

Erdoes A et al., Contribution to the pharmacology and toxicology of various extracts as well as of harpagoside from Harpagophytum procumbens DC, *Planta Med.*, 34:97-108, 1978 *(Chem. Abs.* 90:48368m)

Genazzani E & Sorrentino L, Vascular Action of Acteina: Active Constituent of Actaea racemosa L., *Nature,* 194:544-5, 1962

Gupta MB et al., Anti-inflammatory and Antipyretic Activities of b-Sitosterol, *Planta Med.*, 39:157-63, 1980

Kalashnikova NA & Gerashchenko GI, Antiphlogistic activity of several flavonoids, *Aktual. Vopr. Farm.*, 2:353-4, 1974 *(Chem. Abs.* 84:99345k)

Kenney HE et al., Steroidal Sapogenins. XLVII. Preparation of 16a, 17a-Epoxy-11a-hydroxypregnane-3,20-dione from 5b-Spirostanes, *J. Am. Chem. Soc.*, 80:5568-70, 1958

Kikuchi T et al., New Iridoid Glucosides from Harpagophytum procumbens DC, *Chem. Pharm. Bull.*, 31:2296-2301, 1983

Marker RE et al., Steroidal Sapogenins, *J. Am. Chem. Soc.*, 69:2167-2230, 1947

Piancatelli G, New triterpenes from Actaea racemosa. IV., *Gazz. Chim. Ital.*, 101:139-48, 1971 *(Chem. Abs.* 75:59763c)

Pkheidze TA, Steroidal sapogenins of yuccas growing on the Black Sea coast in Caucasus, *Izv. Akad. Nauk. Gruz. SSR, Ser. Khim.*, 6:309-13, 1980 *(Chem. Abs.* 94:188645g)

Racz-Dotilla E et al., The Action of Taraxacum officinale Extracts on the Body Weight and Diuresis of Laboratory Animals, *Planta Med.*, 26:212-7, 1974

Radics L et al., Carbon-13 NMR Spectra of Some Polycyclic Triterpenoids, *Tetrahed. Lett.*, (48):4287-90, 1975

Roshchin YV & Gerashchenko GI, Antiinflammatory activity of some flavonoids, *Vopr. Farm. Dal'nem Vostoke*, 1:134-5, 1973 *(Chem. Abs.* 83:37683q)

Schindler H, Die Inhaltsstoffe von Heilpflanzen und Prufungsmethoden fur plfanzliche Tinkturen, *Arzneim.-Forsch.*, 2:547-9, 1952

Suntry Ltd., Sodium 3-(a-L-arabinopyranosyl)-16,23-dihydroxyolean-12-en-28-oate, *Chem. Abs.*, 101:322, 1984 (#43572j)

Susnik F, The present state of knowledge about the medicinal plant Taraxacum officinale Weber, *Med. Razgl.*, 21:323-8, 1982

Takanashi M & Mitsuhashi T, Lipid components of the flowers from two species (Taraxacum officinale and Inula cillalis) of the Chrysanthemum family, *Yukagaku*, 22:269-71, 1973 *(Chem. Abs.* 79:63517a)

Wall ME et al., Steroidal Sapogenins VII. Survey of Plants for Steroidal Sapogenins and Other Constituents, *J. Am. Pharm. Assoc.*, 43:1-6, 1954

Westerman L & Roddick JG, Annual Variation in Sterol Levels in Leaves of Taraxacum officinale Weber, *Plant Physiol.*, 68:872-5, 1981

IX SURFACE INFECTIONS

Antifungal and Antiyeast Formula

Acharya RN & Chaubal MG, Essential Oil of Anemopsis californica, *J. Pharm. Sci.*, 57:1020-2, 1968

Ascorbe FJ, The inhibitory action of organic chemicals on a blue stain fungus, *Caribbean Forester*, 14:136-9, 1953 *(Chem. Abs.* 48:12225c)

Clark AM et al., Antimicrobial Activity of Juglone, *Phytother. Res.*, 4:11-4, 1990

Dentali SJ & Hoffmann JJ, Potential Antiinfective Agents from Eriodictyon angustifolium and Salvia apiana, *Int. J. Pharmacognosy*, 30:223-31, 1992

De Oliveira, AB et al., Chemical structures and biological activities of naphthoquinones from Brazilian Bignoniaceae, *Quim. Nova*, 13:302-7, 1990 *(Chem. Abs.* 115:155037j)

Didry N et al., Antimicrobial activity of some naphtoquinones found in plants, *Ann. Pharm. Fr.*, 44:73-8, 1985

Gibaja Oviedo S & Carrillo CG, Chemistry of lichens. II. Study of Usnea barbata (L) Wigg., *Bol. Soc. Quin. Peru,* 50:88-90, 1984 *(Chem. Abs.* 102:109836c)

Girard M et al., Naphthoquinone constituents of Tabebuia spp., *J. Nat. Prod.,* 51:1023-4, 1988

Ikekawa T et al., Isolation and Identification of the Antifungal Active Substance in Walnuts, *Chem. Pharm. Bull.,* 15:242-5, 1967

Joshi KC et al., Quinones and Other Constituents from Tabebuia rosea, *Phytochem.,* 12:942-3, 1973

Kellner W & Kober W, The Possibility of using Ethereal Oils for the Disinfection of Rooms, *Arzneim.-Forsch.,* 5:224-9, 1955

Kligman AM & Rosensweig W, Studies with New Fungistatic Agents I. For the Treatment of Superficial Mycoses, *J. Invest. Derm.,* 10:59-68, 1948

Kurita N et al., Antifungal Activity of Components of Essential Oils, *Agric. Biol. Chem.,* 45:945-52, 1981

Lagrota MHC et al., Antiviral activity of lapachol, *Rev. Microbiol.,* 14:21-6, 1983 *(Chem. Abs.* 99:98871b)

Lee KC & Campbell RW, Nature and Occurrence of Juglone in Juglans nigra L., *HortSci.,* 4:297-8, 1969

de Lima OG et al., First observations on the antimicrobial action of lapachol., *Anais. Soc. Biol. Pernambuco,* 14:129-35, 1956 *(Chem. Abs.* 54:13248i)

de Lima OG et al., A new antibiotic substance isolated from Pau d'Arco (Tabebuia), *Anais. Soc. Biol. Pernambuco,* 14:136-40, 1956 *(Chem. Abs.* 54:13539f)

de Lima OG et al., Antibiotic substances in higher plants. XX. Antimicrobial activity of some derivatives of lapachol as compared with xyloidone, a new natural o-naphthoquinone isolated from extracts of heartwood of Tabebuia avellanedae, *Rev. Inst. Antibiot., Univ. Redife,* 4:3-17, 1962 *(Chem. Abs.* 60:9099g)

de Lima OG et al., Antimicrobial compounds from higher plants. XXXV. Antimicrobial and antitumor activity of lawsone (2-hydroxy-1,4-naphthoquinone) compared with that of lapachol (2-hydroxy-3-(3-methyl-2-butenyl)-1,4-naphthoquinone), *Rev. Inst. Antibiot., Univ. Fed. Pernambuco, Recife,* 11:21-6, 1971 *(Chem. Abs.* 77:29629n)

Maruzzella JC et al., Effects of Vapors of Aromatic Chemicals on Fungi, *J. Pharm. Sci.,* 50:665-8, 1961

Morris JA et al., Antimicrobial Activity of Aroma Chemicals and Essential Oils, *J. Am. Oil Chem. Soc.,* 56:595-603, 1979

Oga S & Sekino T, Toxicity and antiinflammatory activity of Tabebuia avellanedae extracts, *Rev. Fac. Farm. Bioquim. Univ. Sao Paulo*, 7:47-53, 1969

Ohmoto T & Sung YI, Antimycotic substances in the crude drugs. II., *Shoyaku. Zasshi,* 36:307-14, 1982 (*Chem Abs.* 98:204263w)

Otsuka H et al., Antiinflammatory drugs. Antiinflammatory activity of crude drugs and plants. II., *Takeda Kenk. Ho,* 31:247-54, 1972 (*Chem. Abs.* 77:111574z)

Paredes C. A & Arteaga F. M, Extraction of lapachol from Tabebuia species (guayacan), *Politecnica,* 3:163-81, 1975 (*Chem. Abs.* 88:41585e)

Rein BI et al., Antimicrobial action of juglone and its derivatives, *Tr. Kishinev. Sel'sko Khoz. Inst.,* 43:203-13, 1966 (*Chem. Abs.,* 67:106182j)

Reyes Q. A et al., Usnic acid and atranorin in some regional lichens, *Rev. Latinoam. Quim.,* 12:130-1, 1981 (*Chem. Abs.* 96:139704h)

Sturdik E et al., Mechanism of antiyeast activity of juglone, a naturally occuring 1,4-naphthoquinone, *Biologia (Bratislava),* 38:343-51, 1983 (*Chem. Abs.* 99:67412y)

Take Y et al., Role of the Naphthoquinone Moiety in the Biological Activities of Sakyomicin A, *J. Antibiot.,* 39:557-63, 1986

Tripathi RD et al., Structure Activity Relationship amongst Some Fungi toxic a-Naphthoquinones of Angiosperm Origin, *Agric. Biol. Chem.,* 44:2483-5, 1980

Tul'chinskaya VP et al., Effect of compounds from higher plants on the extracellular form and replication of RNA and DNA viruses, *Tr. S'exda Mikrobiol. Ukr., 4th,* pp. 226-7, 1975 (*Chem. Abs.* 86:595y)

Vartia KO, Antibiotics in lichen, *Ann. Med. Exptl. et Biol. Fenniae,* 27:46-54, 1949 (*Chem. Abs.* 43:5077a)

Vidal-Tessier AM et al., Lipophilic quinones of the trunk wood of Tabebuia serratifolia (Vahl.) Nichols, *Ann. Pharm. Fr.,* 46:55-7, 1988 (*Chem. Abs.* 109:208265s)

Antiseptic Formula

Amin AH et al., Berberine sulfate: antimicrobial activity, bioassay, and mode of action, *Can. J. Microbiol.,* 15:1067-76, 1969

Babbar OP et al., Effect of berberine chloride eye drops on clinically positive trachoma patients, *Indian J. Med. Res.,* 76(Suppl):83-8, 1982

Bauer R et al., Immunological in vivo and in vitro Examinations of Echinacea Extracts, *Arzneim.-Forsch.,* 38:276-281, 1988

Bauer R et al., TLC and HPLC Analysis of Echinacea pallida and E. angustifolia Roots, *Planta Med.,* 54:426-30, 1988

Bauer R et al., Alkamides from the Roots of Echinacea angustifolia, *Phytochem.*, 28:505-8, 1989

Genest K & Hughes DW, Natural Products in Canadian Pharmaceuticals IV. Hydrastis Canadensis, *Can. J. Pharm. Sci.*, 4:41-5, 1969

Ghosh AK et al., Effect of berberine chloride on Leishmania donovani, *Indian J. Med. Res.*, pp. 407-16, 1983

Guandalini S et al., Effects of berberine on basal and secretagogue-modified ion transport in the rabbit ileum in vitro, *J. Pediatr. Gastroenterol. Nutr.*, 6:953-60, 1987

Gupte S, Use of Berberine in Treatment of Giardiasis, *Am. J. Dis. Child.*, 129:866, 1975

Hocking GM, Echinacea Angustifolia (Cone Flower) as Crude Drug, *Quart. J. Crude Drug Res.*, 5:679-83, 1965

Johnson CC et al., Toxicity of Alkaloids to Certain Bacteria. II. Berberine, Physostigmine, and Sanguinarine, *Acta Pharmacol. Toxicol.*, 8:71-8, 1952

Kaiser E & Winkler G, The Problem of Competitive Inhibition in the Enzymatic System of Hyaluronic Acid and Hyaluronidase, *Arzneim.-Forsch.*, 5:322-4, 1955

Lahiri SC & Dutta NK, Berberine and Chloramphenicol in the Treatment of Cholera and Severe Diarrhoea, *J. Indian Med. Assoc.*, 48:1-11, 1967

Mahajan VM et al., Antimycotic Activity of Berberine Sulphate: An Alkaloid from an Indian Medicinal Herb, *Sabouraudia*, 20:79-81, 1982

Mirska I et al., Effect of berberine sulfate on healthy mice infected with Candida albicans, *Arch. Immunol. Ther. Exp.*, 20:921-9, 1972 (*Chem. Abs.* 78:79761r)

Otsuka H et al., Studies on anti-inflammatory agents. II. Anti-inflammatory constituents from rhizome of Coptis japonica Makino, *Yaku. Zasshi,* 101:883-90, 1981 (*Chem. Abs.* 96:28395p)

Poe CF & Johnson CC, Toxicity of Hydrastine, Hydrastinine, and Sparteine, *Acta Pharmacol. Toxicol.*, 10:338-46, 1954

Potopal'skii AI et al., Antimicrobic and antineoplastic properties of alkaloids of greater celandine and their thiophosphamide derivatives, *Mikrobiol. Zh. (Kiev)*, 37:755-9, 1975

Rabbani GH et al., Randomized Controlled Trial of Berberine Sulfate Therapy for Diarrhea Due to Enterotoxigenic Escherichia coli and Vibrio cholerae, *J. Infect. Dis.*, 155:979-84, 1987

Reisch J et al., The Problem of the Microbiological Activity of Simple Acetylene Compounds, *Arzneim.-Forsch.*, 17:816-25, 1967

Sack RB & Froehlich JL, Berberine Inhibits Intestinal Secretory Response of Vibrio cholerae and Escherichia coli Enterotoxins, *Infect. Immun.*, 35:471-5, 1982

Schein FT & Hanna C, The absorption, distribution, and excretion of berberine, *Arch. Intern. Pharmacodynamie,* 124:317-25, 1960 (*Chem. Abs.* 54:14473e)

Schulte KE et al., The Presence of Polyacetylene Compounds in Echinacea purpurea Mnch. and Echinacea angustifolia DC, *Arzneim.-Forsch.,* 17:825-9, 1967

Sharda DC, Berberine in the Treatment of Diarrhoea of Infancy and Childhood, *J. Indian Med. Assoc.,* 54:22-4, 1970

Stoll A et al., Isolierung und Konstitution des Echinacosids, eines Glykosids aus den Wurzeln von Echinacea angustifolia D.C., *Helv. Chim. Acta,* 33:1877-93, 1950

Subbaiah TV & Amin AH, Effect of Berberine Sulphate on Entamoeba histolytica, *Nature,* 215:527-8, 1967

Sun D et al., Influence of berberine sulfate on synthesis and expression of Pap fimbrial adhesin in uropathogenic Escherichia coli, *Antimicrob. Agents Chemother.,* 32:1274-7, 1988

Sun D et al., Berberine sulfate blocks adherence of Streptococcus pyogenes to epithelial cells, fibronectin, and hexadecane, *Antimicrob. Agents Chemother.,* 32:1370-4, 1988

Tai Y-H et al., Antisecretory effects of berberine in rat ileum, *Am. J. Physiol.,* 241:G253-8, 1981

Tragni E et al., Evidence from Two Classic Irritation Tests for an Anti-inflammatory Action of a Natural Extract, Echinacina B, *Fd. Chem. Toxic.,* 23:317-9, 1985

Tragni E et al., Anti-Inflammatory Activity of Echinacea angustifolia Fractions Separated on The Basis of Molecular Weight, *Pharmacol. Res. Comm.,* 20:(Suppl. V):87-90, 1988

Tubaro A et al., Anti-inflammatory activity of a polysaccharidic fraction of Echinacea angustifolia, *J. Pharm. Pharmacol.,* 567-9, 1987

Wagner H et al., Immunostimulating Polysaccharides (Heteroglycans) of Higher Plants, *Arzneim.-Forsch.,* 35:1069-75, 1985

Zhu B & Ahrens FA, Effect of berberine on intestinal secretion mediated by Escherichia coli heat-stable enterotoxin in jejunum of pigs, *Am. J. Vet. Res.,* 43:1594-8, 1982

Ear Canal Formula

Adetumbi MA & Lau BHS, Allium Sativum (Garlic) - A Natural Antibiotic, *Med. Hypoth.,* 12:227-37, 1983

Barone FE & Tansey MR, Isolation, Purification, Identification, Synthesis, and Kinetics of Activity of the Anticandidal Component of Allium sativum, and a Hypothesis for its Mode of Action, *Mycologia,* 69:793-825, 1977

Brantner A & Brantner H, Screening of Flavonoid Aglycones and Glycosides for Antimicrobial Activity, *Planta Med.*, 57(Suppl.2):A43, 1991

Bystrov NS et al., The Structure of Hyperforin, *Tetrahed. Lett.*, 32:2791-4,
1975

Gaind KN & Ganjoo TN, Antibacterial Principle of Hypericum
perforatum Linn., *Indian J. Pharm.*, 21:172-5, 1959

Ghannoum MA, Studies on the Anticandidal Mode of Action of Allium
sativum (Garlic), *J. Gen. Microbiol.*, 134:2917-24, 1988

Gurevich AI et al., Hyperforin, an antibiotic from Hypericum perforatum,
Antibiotiki (Moscow), 16:510-3, 1971 *(Chem. Abs.* 75:95625t)

Hoelzl J & Ostrowski E, St. John's wort (Hypericum perforatum L.).
HPLC analysis of the main components and their variability in a
population, *Dtsch. Apoth. Ztg.*, 127:1227-30, 1987 *(Chem. Abs.*
107:112686n)

Hudson JB et at., Antiviral activities of hypericin, *Antiviral Res.*, 15:101-
12, 1991

Hughes BG & Lawson LD, Antimicrobial Effects of Allium sativum L.
(Garlic), Allium ampeloprasum L. (Elephant Garlic), and Allium cepa
L. (Onion), Garlic Compounds and Commercial Garlic Supplement
Products, *Phytother. Res.*, 5:1548, 1991

Kalashnikova NA & Gerashchenko GI, Antiphlogistic activity of several
flavonoids, *Aktual. Vopr. Farm.*, 2:353-4, 1974 *(Chem. Abs.*
84:99346m)

Kraus GA et al., Antiretroviral Activity of Synthetic Hypericin and
Related Analogs, *Biochem. Biophys. Res. Comm.*, 172:149-53, 1990

Kraus J & Franz G, Mucilage polysaccharide from mullein flowers, *Dtsch.
Apoth. Ztg.*, 127:665-9, 1987 *(Chem. Abs.* 106:211001w)

Lavie G et al., Studies of the mechanisms of action of the antiretroviral
agents hypericin and pseudohypericin, *Proc. Natl. Acad. Sci. U.S.A.*,
86:5963-7, 1989 *(Chem. Abs.* 111:126513y)

Meruelo D et al., Therapeutic agents with dramatic antiretroviral activity
and little toxicity at effective doses: Aromatic polycyclic diones
hypericin and pseudohypericin, *Proc. Natl. Acad. Sci. U.S.A.*,
85:5230-4, 1988

Negrash AK & Pochinok PY, Comparative study of chemotherapeutic and
pharmacological properties of antimicrobial preparations from
common St. John's wort, *Fitontsidy, Mater. Soveshch., 6th*, pp. 198-
200, 1972

Skwarek T, Effects of some vegetable preparations on propagation of the
influenza viruses. I. Effects of vegetable preparations on propagation
of the influenza viruses in cultures of chicken embryo fibroblasts and

in chicken embryos, *Acta Pol. Pharm.*, 36:605-12, 1979 *(Chem. Abs.* 93:37018h)

Skwarek T, Effect of some vegetable preparations on propagation of the influenza viruses. II. Attempts at interferon induction, *Acta Pol. Pharm.*, 36:715-20, 1979 *(Chem. Abs.* 93:37020c)

Souleles C & Geronikaki A, Flavonoids from Verbascum thapsus, *Sci. Pharm.*, 57:59-61, 1989 *(Chem. Abs.* 111:83947y)

Takahashi I et al., Hypericin and Pseudohypericin Specifically Inhibit Protein Kinase C: Possible Relation to their Antiretroviral Activity, *Biochem. Biophys. Res. Comm.*, 165:1207-12, 1989

Tang J et al., Virucidal activity of hypericin against enveloped and non-enveloped DNA and RNA viruses, *Antiviral Res.*, 13:313-25, 1990

Vanden Berghe DA et al., Present Status and Prospects of Plant Products as Antiviral Agents, *Adv. Med. Plant Res.*, pp. 47-99, 1985

Vasil'chenka EA et al., Analgesic action of Flavonoids of Rhododendron luteum Sweet, Hypericum perforatum L., Lespedeza bicolor Turoz. and L. hedysaroides (Pall.) Kitag., *Rastit. Resur.*, 22:12-21, 1986 *(Chem. Abs.* 104:142140k)

Yamada Y & Azuma K, Evaluation of the In Vitro Antifungal Activity of Allicin, *Anticicrob. Agents Chemother.*, 11:743-9, 1977

GLOSSARY

acupuncture - a method of treating conditions by inserting needles into specific points on the body to influence energy flow

adaptogens - nontoxic tonic agents whose nonspecific effects help to normalize physiologic activity

adrenergic - autonomic nerves stimulated by adrenalin (epinephrine) and norepinephrinewhich activate the "fright, flight, or fight" reaction by increasing heart rate, breathing, and blood flow to skeletal muscles

aglycone - the portion of a glycoside with the sugar component removed

alimentary - pertaining to digestion and digestive organs, particularly the tract from the mouth to the anus

alkaloids - basic, physiologically-active, nitrogen-containing plant constituents with a bitter taste

alteratives - agents that improve the removal of wastes from the circulation and enhance their excretion

anthelmintics - agents that weaken, paralyze (vermifuges) or kill (vermicides) worms

anti-inflammatory - an agent that ameliorates conditions characterized by redness, pain, heat, swelling, and loss of function

antilithics - agents that prevent the formation and/or aggregation of crystalline compounds

antimicrobial - antiseptic; an agent that kills or inhibits the growth of microorganisms

antispasmodic - an agent that reduces strong, involuntary muscular contractions

antitussive - reduces the tendency to cough

aromatics - essential oils; fragrant, volatile oil con stituents of plants

astringents - agents that have a local contracting effect on the surface of tissues

autonomic - the system that regulates unconscious organ functions and includes adrenergic (sympathetic) and cholinergic (parasympathetic) nerves

biofeedback - the use of mechanical devices to measure autonomic functions and alert the user of physiologic changes produced by exerting a conscious influence

bronchodilators - agents that widen the air passages (inside the bronchial tubes) of the lungs

carminatives - aromatic agents that relieve spasms in the intestines and aid in the expulsion of gas

cathartics - purgatives; agents that cause a strong, rapid evacuation of the bowels

chiropractic - a system of assessing and manually treating conditions based on nerve function and the alignment of the spine

cholagogues - agents that increase the flow of bile into the small intestine

choleretics - agents that increase the production of bile by the liver

cholinergic - autonomic nerves stimulated by acetylcholine which activate digestion and elimination

constituents - components; compounds that are contained in a plant or extract

demulcents - bland agents that sooth surface irritations by their coating effect

diaphoretics - agents that increase perspiration

diuretics - agents that increase urinary output

eclectic - incorporates the use of diverse approaches, especially the most effective therapeutic practices

empirical - use based on experience

emunctories - organs that excrete waste products

found in the fluids of the body

expectorants - agents that promotes expulsion of mucus from the air passages of the lungs

febrifuge - an agent that reduces fevers

flavonoids - bioactive constituents often seen as pigments in plants that contain oxygen in multiple cyclic molecules

glycosides - plant constituents consisting of a sugar molecule bound to a nonsugar component

herbalism - the use of remedies of plant origin to help promote or regain health

holistic - an approach that addresses the interrelated functions of the entire person and involves the influence of the body, mind, and spirit on healing

homeopathy - a system of medicine that uses minute doses of substances to treat symptoms that those same substances cause in a healthy person

hydrotherapy - the use of water to produce therapeutic effects to the body, mainly through local tissue reactions to its temperature and/or pressure

hygienics - the therapeutic system advocating proper lifestyle, diet, and elimination to promote health

hypnotherapy - the therapeutic application of suggestions or commands to someone in an induced, passive, receptive state

immune - resistant to disease because of antibody, white blood cell, and other defensive responses to foreign substances, mutations, and microorganisms

laxatives - agents that mildly stimulate the evacuation of the bowels

lymph - fluid outside of the blood vessels and tissue cells in the body

metabolism - organized chemical changes that build up or breakdown substances to maintain life

microorganisms - microbes; microscopic life-forms

such as viruses, bacteria, yeast, and protozoa

mucosa - the mucus-secreting membrane covering the inner surface of organ tracts and ducts

National Formulary - a book that describes prepara tions officially recognized as medicines in the United States that are not included in the *United States Pharmacopeia*

naturopathy - a system of medicine that utilizes natural substances, forces, and methods to in crease vitality and support the healing power of nature

nervine - agents that have a calming or modifying influence on central nervous system functions

neurotransmitter - a physiologic substance that stimulates a nerve to pass on an impulse

osteopathy - a system of medicine emphasizing the importance of normal body mechanics and utilizing manipulative methods of correcting faulty structure

phagocytosis - the ingestion of microorganisms, cells, and foreign particles by specialized white blood cells and tissue cells

physiologic - part of the body's normal system of functioning

physiomedicalism - a system of medicine that utilizes primarily nontoxic herbs as remedies

physiotherapy - the therapeutic use of physical agents and methods such as water, movements, massage, and energy forms including heat, cold, light, electricity, and ultrasound

phytoestrogens - plant components that have estro-gen activity in animals

polysaccharides - constituents that consist of numer-ous sugars, often of varying types, bonded together

purgatives - see *cathartics*

saponins - glycoside constituents of plants consisting of a sapogenin bound to a sugar that form a foam when shaken in water

sedatives - agents that allay excitement or activity, especially of the nervous system

stimulants - agents that acts to excite an organ or system to functional activity

stomachics - bitter substances that promote the functional activity of the stomach

synergistic - enhancing; the influence that occurs when one compound combined with another produces an effect that is greater than their individual activities added together

tannins - water-soluble, astringent constituents of plants

teas - water extracts of plant parts made either by soaking at room temperature (cold infusions) or in hot water (infusions) or by boiling (decoctions)

terpenes - hydrocarbon plant constituents characterized by their aromatic properties

tinctures - liquid remedies that contain distilled alcohol and water as solvents

tonics - agents that restore the tone or activity of an organ or system that is not functioning optimally

vasodilators - agents that increase blood flow to a part by widening the caliber of arterial blood vessels

vehicles - substances, usually liquid, to which a remedy is added that makes the remedy easier to use

vulnerary - an agent that promotes the healing of wounds

INDEX OF HERBS & FORMULAS

FRANCIS BRINKER. N.D.

Francis Brinker, N.D., is a 1981 graduate of the National College of Naturopathic Medicine in Portland, Oregon. In addition, he completed the two year Postgraduate Studies Program in Botanical Medicine and taught Botanical Medicine at the National College of Naturopathic Medicine until 1985.

Dr. Brinker's undergraduate work includes a Bachelor of Science Degree in Human Biology from Kansas Newman College and a Bachelor of Arts Degree in Biology from the University of Kansas, Phi Beta Kappa.

He is currently an instructor at the Southwest College of Naturopathic Medicine and Health Sciences and a researcher of historic, scientific and medical literature.

In addition to numerous articles published in European and U.S. professional journals, Dr. Brinker is author of *The Eclectic Dispensatory of Botanical Therapeutics, Vol. II,* and a major contributor to *The Eclectic Dispensatory of Botanical Therapeutics, Vol. I.* His work, *The Toxicology of Botanical Medicine,* is available through Eclectic Medical Publications and is recognized as the finest study of medicinal plant toxicology currently available.

Also Available From Eclectic Medical Publications

Lectures In Naturopathic Hydrotherapy
Andre Saine, N.D. and Wade Boyle, N.D.
Hydrotherapies enhance the body's immune response, improve cellular
nutrition and detoxify. This work gives detailed guidance for thirteen
hydrotherapy treatments. Excellent for health practitioners, homeopaths
and lay persons interested in a safe but powerful healing tool.
1988   235 pages $35.00

Reading The Eye, Pulse And Tongue For The Indicated Remedy
Wade Boyle, N.D., Editor
A series of articles written 75 years ago by Eli Jones, M.D., for the
Homeopathic Recorder, this work explains how findings from physical
examination enable appropriate remedy selection. Emphasis is on botanical medicines with methodology credit given to homeopathy and
biochemic expounder, Shuessler.
1989   95 pages $15.00

**Herb Doctors: Pioneers In Ninetenth Century American Botanical
Medicine And A History Of The Eclectic Medical Institute**
Wade Boyle, N.D.
Well researched, referenced and indexed. Offers an accurate and detailed
understanding of America's rich heritage of herbal medicine. Includes a
history of the Eclectic Medical Institute of Cincinnati, Ohio, and bio-
graphical portraits of the great doctors of the time.
1988   66 pages $15.00

**Official Herbs: Botanical Substances In The United States
Pharmacopoeias, 1820-1990**
Wade Boyle, N.D.
For anyone interested in medicinal plants and their former official status as
medicines in the United States.
1991   77 pages $20.00

Nature Doctors
Friedhelm Kirchfeld and Wade Boyle, N.D.
Part I focuses on pivotal figures of the European nature cure movement,
almost all of whom discovered their approaches in response to their own
"incurable" illnesses. Part II is devoted to doctors who established
naturopathy in America: Benedict and Louisa Lust, Henry Lindlahr, Otis
Carroll, John Bastyr, etc. Inspiring and informative for modern holistic
medicine enthusiasts.
1994   335 pages $29.95

Eclectic Medical Publications P.O. Box 936 Sandy, OR 97055
1-800-865-1487